Mediterranean Diet Cookbook

The Complete Guide Solution With Meal Plan And Recipes For Weight Loss, Gain Energy And Fat Burn With Recipes And Essential Fat Loss Recipes For The Ultimate Healthy Lifestyle

Jimmy Morris

Published by Jason Thawne Publishing House

© Jimmy Morris

Mediterranean Diet Cookbook: The Complete Guide Solution With Meal Plan And Recipes For Weight Loss, Gain Energy And Fat Burn With Recipes And Essential Fat Loss Recipes For The Ultimate Healthy Lifestyle

All Rights Reserved

ISBN 978-1-989749-86-9

This document is geared towards providing exact and reliable information in regards to the topic and issue covered. The publication is sold with the idea that the publisher isn't required to render accounting, officially permitted, or otherwise, qualified services. If advice is necessary, legal or even professional, a practiced individual in the profession should be ordered.

- From a Declaration of Principles which was accepted and approved equally by a Committee of the American Bar Association and a Committee of Publishers and Associations.

In no way is it legal to reproduce, duplicate, or even transmit any part of this document in either electronic means or in printed format. Recording of this publication is strictly prohibited and any storage of this document isn't allowed unless with proper written permission from the publisher. All rights reserved.

The information provided herein is stated to be truthful and consistent, in that any liability, in terms of inattention or otherwise, by any usage or abuse of any policies, processes, or directions contained within is the solitary and also utter responsibility of the recipient reader. Under no circumstances will any legal responsibility or blame be held against the publisher for any reparation, damages, or monetary loss due to the information herein, either directly or indirectly.

Respective authors own all copyrights not held by the publisher.

The information herein is offered for just informational purposes solely, and is universal as so. The presentation of the information is without contract or any type of guarantee assurance.

The trademarks that are used are without any consent, and also the publication of the trademark is without permission or backing by the trademark owner. All trademarks and brands within this book are for clarifying purposes only and are the owned by the owners themselves, not affiliated with this document.

TABLE OF CONTENTS

Part 1 1

Introduction: Smooth All The Way 10

Chapter One: Mediterranean Diet 5

Chapter Two: Foods In The Diet 8

Chapter Three: Main Courses............................ 11

Mediterranean Recipes...................................... 11

Filet Mignon 11

Pork Tenderloin With Apple Succotash 13

Crostini With Buffalo Mozzarella, Peppers & Basil 14

Mushroom, Macaroni Tuna Dish....................... 15

Chapter Four: Chicken & Couscous Soup........... 16

Simple Soba Noodle Soup 17

Veggie Laksa 18

Zucchini (Courgette) Soup................................. 19

Pea & Pasta Soup With Bacon 20

Chapter Five: Salads And Vegetables 22

Classic To Dress Peppery Wild Rocket 22

Broccoli With Chickpeas & Tahini Sauce........... 23

Wilted Green With Parmesan 24

Field Mushrooms With Feta & Olive Dressing ... 25

Mushroom, Macaroni Tuna Dish 27

Macaroni Cheese 27

Chicken Or Veal Scaloppini................................ 28

Chicken With Onion Sauce 30

Chapter Six: Meat Balls With Sweet And Sour Sauce 32

Left Over Meat 33

Meat Loaf 35

Hot Tuna Fritters.. 36

Chicken In Onion Sauce..................................... 37

Chicken Cacciatore.. 37

Part 2 46

Introduction... 47

Chapter 1: What Is The Mediterranean Diet?.... 49

What To Eat: 51

What To Eat In Moderation: 52

Rarely Eat: *Red Meat* 52

Avoid These Foods:... 52

Essential Nutrients.. 55

Tips Of How To Reap The Benefits 55

Chapter 2: Breakfast Recipes 57

Breakfast Couscous... 57

Banana Nut Oatmeal 58

Mediterranean Breakfast Quinoa 59

Almond Biscotti 60

Mediterranean Slices 61

Avocado Egg Salad 63

Mediterranean Eggs On Toast 63

Potato Hash And Chickpeas 65

Chapter 3: Lunch Recipes 67

Two-Bean Greek Salad 67

Greek Avocado Salad 68

Garden Wraps 70

Creamy Paninis 72

Chicken Souvlaki With Tzatziki 73

Shrimp Pasta 75

Scampi Greek-Style 76

Salmon With Slaw 78

Lamb With Garlic & Rosemary 80

Broad Bean And Feta Cheese Toasts 81

Rigatoni With Asiago Cheese & Green Olive-Almond Pesto 83

Mediterranean Quinoa Salad 84

Broiled Feta With Olives & Roasted Peppers 86

Brussels Sprouts With Honey Pomegranate And Apples... 88

Chapter 4: Dinner Recipes................................. 91

Stuffed Grape Leaves Casserole 93

Grilled Chicken With Quinoa Greek Salad 95

Grilled Chicken And Grape Skewers 97

Lemon-Zaatar-Grilled Chicken........................... 99

Easy & Quick Gyros With Tzatziki Sauce 100

Chicken Kofte & Zucchini 101

Grilled Lamb Chops And Mint 103

Hummus Turkey Sliders 105

Beef Steaks Crusted In Cumin With Olive-Orange Relish.. 107

Kofte In A Hurry 108

Chickpea Patties 110

Lemon Salmon And Lima Beans 112

Bass With Mushrooms And Spaghetti Squash . 114

Mussels With Olives And Potatoes.................. 118

Seared Tuna Steaks... 120

Mushroom Kabobs 121

Mediterranean Potato Salad 123

Roasted Peppers—Anchovies—And Tomatoes 124

Herbed Mashed Potatoes With Greek Yogurt . 125

Egg & Lemon Greek Soup................................ 127

Chapter 5: Dessert And Snack Recipes 128

Ricotta Cheesecake.. 129

Almond Cake 129

Traditional Greek Yogurt Cake In Syrup........... 131

Grape Harvest Cake 133

Almond Coffee Cookies.................................... 135

Chocolate Chip-Oatmeal Raisin Cookies.......... 136

Cucumber Roll Ups 137

Pita Pizzas And Hummus.................................. 138

Mediterranean Skewers With Bloody Mary Vinaigrette... 140

Cranberry, Goat Cheese, And Walnut Canapés 142

Greek Yogurt Parfait 143

Yogurt And Honey With Walnuts: Greek-Style 145

Lemon Cream & Blueberries 145

Chapter 6: Continue The Plan 147

Sample Meal Plan 147

Healthy Snacks... 149

How To Eat Out And Remain On The Diet 150

The Substitution List 150

Conclusion .... **ERROR! BOOKMARK NOT DEFINED.**

Conclusion 153

About The Author 153

Part 1

INTRODUCTION: SMOOTH ALL THE WAY

It's a truth that all humanity eat to live. That is a fact that cannot be denied or refuted, but there are some people who also live to eat. It is a choice that we all have to make in this life. Lovers of food and different cuisines from all over the world expend significant amounts of time and energy in search of different diets. Therefore Vitality of Mediterranean Diets is a book that serves to inform us about the region of this diverse place and the different recipes that are offered there. It is refreshing for people in other parts of the world to know that these recipes are life-enhancing and can be prepared in other parts of the world.

Vitality of Mediterranean Diets deals with diets from the Mediterranean region. It offers several recipes of foods, from different ways to cook and present meats and fish to salads and desserts and appetisers. If you have recently decided to try out cuisines from different regions, perhaps because you are bored of eating the same dishes, then this book has something for you. If you are a foodie, and you have always had the urge to sample what other cultures and regions across the world eat, then this book provides many recipes indigenous to the Mediterranean region that offer a wide range of tastes guaranteed to provide different sensations. The maxim, diversity is the spice of life aptly applies here and if you can give the recipes incorporated in this book a try, then disappointment will be a far away frustration. Even if you just like cooking something different once in a while, whether it is for a party or a get-together of you and your friends, or even if you are a professional chef and are looking for new recipes to excite and tantalise your clients, this book is a must have in your arsenal of recipes.

This book will:

☐ Offer you several recipes to choose from; different ways to cook food that gives it an exotic Mediterranean flair.

☐ Give you tips on healthy recipes that are delicious and still good for your body and your lifestyle.

☐Inform you on the benefits of each recipe in it, outlining the health advantages of the recipes and the recommended portions.

☐It will demystify the notion that these recipes are beyond rich of people in other parts of the world.

☐The choice of what recipe one wants to adapt is as diverse as the region itself. This book thus becomes a one-shop stop that will minimize the rigors of going to look for diets.

I therefore welcome aboard The Vitality of Mediterranean Diets for your sampling that will provoke you to adapt them as your cherished recipes. Remember the world has become a global village and therefore you cannot remain in the dark places of dietary retrogression while the world is moving forward. I have taken my time to package this book for you and I believe it will be the gem that you have been looking for to beef up your health as a recipe enthusiast.

CHAPTER ONE: MEDITERRANEAN DIET

It's a diet of the inhabitants residing in places around the Mediterranean region. Nations around these areas have a rich culture and food history. These nations have all contributed to the making of these mouth-watering cuisines. The nutrition benefits go beyond one's imagination. Talk of the all round olive oil and the rich protein giving legumes. The fish and the wine are so enthralling to all and sundry. These foods help reduce the chances of a person getting high blood pressure and cancer once a person creates a routine out of them.

A hallmark of Mediterranean dishes is that they derive deep flavour from simple ingredients. Less time is spent in the kitchen. Ten minutes in the kitchen leaves more time for the activities and people you love. It's hard to choose just one menu, but here's what a day's worth of meals might be. For breakfast, Greek yogurt topped with berries and walnuts will suffice and either coffee or tea.

For lunch, lentil soup with Swiss chard topped with tzatziki sauce is most preferable. One can also top it up with hummus and pita. For snacks, whole grain crackers and cheese will do well to the body. When it comes to the dessert, fresh fruit drizzled with honey gives the body a refreshing feel.

Diet alone can reverse heart disease, stroke and still lower cholesterol without medications. People following a Mediterranean diet can stave off need for diabetes drugs and help prevent other related diseases.

It is a diet that can modify estrogens level and, for this reason, reduce the chances of getting cancer. People from the Mediterranean countries have lower rates of hip fractures or osteoporosis. Fruits have significant role in cognitive capacity and, as a result, counter the risk of getting

Alzheimer. It is a diet that helps to alleviate constipation, irritable bowel syndrome, acid reflux, arthritis, autoimmune diseases, and blindness.

CHAPTER TWO: FOODS IN THE DIET

Eat naturally, unprocessed foods like fruits, vegetables, whole grains and nuts. Make olive oil your primary source of dietary fat. Reduce the consumption of red meat while eating low to moderate amounts of fish per week. Drink a moderate quantity of wine as one or two glasses per day for men and one for women.

Foods to Eat

Make sure you take three to four pieces of fruit every day and see to it that one of the pieces is an orange; they are very high in antioxidants and phytochemicals. These phytochemicals are substances that protect us against diseases. Berries such as strawberries, blueberries, raspberries are also a must in this diet because of their antioxidants elements.

Vegetables

Include also a salad in your primary meals. Use olive oil and lemon for dressing since this is a powerful antioxidant combination. Tomatoes and tomato products are a staple food in the Mediterranean diet for they contain lycopene while salads complete Mediterranean side dish. Zucchini is also a delightful complement when you fry them in the all-round olive oil.

Olive Oil

Use olive oil in your meals both to cook and as a condiment in your salads. Olive oil is the primary element in these recipes.

Sea Food

Sea food like fish, when eaten two or three times a week proves very essential. Salmon and sardines are excellent choices because they provide omega-3 oils, which are fats that the body needs, but cannot create in enough quantities.

Garlic and Aromatic Herbs

It is good to use garlic and aromatic herbs as condiment. Garlic is the leading contributor to the low incidence of high blood pressure in Mediterranean countries because it dilates the blood vessels walls.

Try to take legumes eight times a week. Legumes are a little fat, and fiber filled and a good source of protein. Limit refined grains and choose whole grains. Lower fat dairy options should replace full-fat milk products. Olive oil would be restricted to a tablespoon per day. The human body requires dietary fat, and plant-based oil to function smoothly.

Take a fruit for dessert and consume no more than two eggs per week. Replace butter with olive oil for cooking. Use honey to sweeten the recipe but do not add sugar. Eat red meats once a month and couple it with a thirty-minute session of moderate physical activity each day.

CHAPTER THREE: MAIN COURSES

Mediterranean Recipes

Filet Mignon

(1)Teaspoonful each of salt and black pepper
(2)Teaspoonful Thyme
(3)Two cloves garlic, chopped
(4)2 Teaspoonful of extra virgin olive oil
(5)Two pounds-Filet Mignon

Mix oil and pepper together and then add salt and thyme into the bowl. Slit the meat several times across and apply the spice concoction on the slits. Place the meat in a fridge. You can now roast this treated meat for about thirty minutes. Finally get the meat from the fridge and allow to cool before serving.

Striped Bass (in a Pouch)

(1)Four pieces of parchment or aluminium foil, 18x18
(2)4-1/2 pound fish fillets

(3)Eight cloves of garlic, crushed; salt and pepper to taste

(4)Four sprigs of fresh thyme

(5)3 lemons

(6)1/2 cup pitted Kalamata olives

(7)One basket of heirloom cherry tomatoes

(8)One can drained artichoke hearts, quartered

(9)One fennel bulb, thinly sliced

(10)1/2 cup white wine

(11)1/4 cup lemon juice

(12)1/4 bunch of chopped Italian parsley

(13)Quarter cup of olive oil

Put all these elements in one bowl. You then add pepper and olive oil and mix and later put vinegar and garlic.

Potato Casserole and Chicken

(1)1 lb. small potatoes (red, white, or purple)

(2)One rotisserie chicken, shredded

(3)1 1/2 T. kosher salt

(4)1 T. Dijon mustard

(5)2 T. white wine vinegar (red wine vinegar is good too)

(6)One t. Honey

(7)One t. Pepper
(8)6 T. olive oil (half the oil works well too)
(9)Two garlic cloves, minced
(10)2 T. capers drained
(11)Two handfuls of spinach leaves.

Prepare potatoes to a point of tenderness for twenty minutes. Put them aside as and cut them in half after they have cooled. In the meantime cut the chicken and put it in a bowl. In a different dish, mix vinegar and mustard as you mix. Then add whisk garlic and honey. When satisfied that all have mixed well, add pepper and salt. On top of the chicken, add spinach leaves and the potatoes that are still hot. This helps to wilting your spinach. Finally you should add the capers as you pour vinaigrette and toss lightly. Serve warm.

Pork Tenderloin with Apple Succotash
(1)Coarse salt
(2)2 T. chilli powder
(3)Two pork tenderloins(about 2 pounds total), trimmed
(4)Olive oil

(5) 1/4 cup vegetable or chicken broth
(6) One 10-oz. Package of frozen baby lima beans
(7) Four ears corn, kernels removed, or 1 frozen package
(8) Two semi-tart apples, peeled and finely chopped
(9) Ground pepper

Crostini with Buffalo Mozzarella, Peppers & Basil

The secret of this recipe is the cheese. Choose buffalo mozzarella but not the ordinary bocconcini. If this cannot be found, then ricotta or goats cheese are an option. Mix with roast peppers and if not, use capsicum.
(1) Eight thin slices baguette
(2) One large ball buffalo mozzarella, torn into chunks roasted & peeled
(3) Cut leaves of basil and those of Capsicum
Toast baguette pieces and add mozzarella chunks. Top these with red pepper and basil leaves.

Mushroom, Macaroni Tuna Dish

(1) One large onion
(2) One can mushroom or celery soup
(3) Pinch mixed herbs ½ cup grated cheese
(4) Grated lemon rind
(5) One can tuna
(6) 1 cup cooked macaroni or rice
(7) ½ cup creamy milk
(8) 2 chopped gherkins

Fry your cut onion as you add milk and soup. It should also include soup while you add tuna. Herbs and gherkins should be added to macaroni and rind. Heat in a dish and add cheese.

CHAPTER FOUR: CHICKEN & COUSCOUS SOUP

Couscous is brilliant in soup as it cooks quickly and adds a lovely hearty texture to make your soup more of a meal-in-a-bowl. If you have access to kale or other greens they may be substituted for the baby spinach for a more rustic soup.

(1) 6 cups chicken stock or broth
(2) 2 chicken breasts, finely sliced into ribbons
(3) 1/2 cup couscous
(4) 2 bags baby spinach, washed
(5) 4-5 tablespoons lemon juice

Bring the stock to the boil in a large saucepan. Add chicken and cook for 2 - 3 minutes or until just cooked through. Scoop the chicken and divide between 4 bowls. Keep warm. Meanwhile return the broth to the boil. Add couscous and return to the boil then stir through the spinach leaves until they are just wilted. Add lemon juice, season and taste. Add a little more lemon juice if you think it needs it.

Divide couscous and spinach broth between the bowls and serve hot.

Simple Soba Noodle Soup

Soba noodles are made of buckwheat as well as regular wheat and have a subtle 'healthy' flavour. Most other noodles could be used here if you prefer. Likewise, the veggies can be varied to suit your taste (and what you have in the fridge!) baby spinach would be lovely. Remember that the noodles are going to keep cooking in the broth after you've served up so best to slightly undercook first.

(1)1 1/2 cups vegetable stock
handful soba noodles (approx 50g or 2oz)
(2) 3 heads baby bok choy, leaves separated
large pinch chilli flakes, optional
(3)1 – 2 tablespoons soy sauce
Bring stock to the boil in a medium saucepan. Add noodles and simmer for 2 minutes. Add bok choy and chilli and 1T soy sauce and simmer for another minute or until noodles are only just cooked (see

note above).Remove from the heat. Taste and add extra soy if needed. Serve hot.

Veggie Laksa

Laksa is a wonderful coconut milk based noodle soup that hails from Malaysia. These days you can get commercial laska or other Thai curry pastes that take all the hard work out of it. Singapore noodles can also be used in this recipe which is a fine version of fresh hokkien noodles. Chicken laksa is also really popular. Prawn or shrimps are lovely cooked in the spicy fragrant coconut broth.

(1)350g (3/4lb) fresh Singapore noodles
(2)60g (2oz) Laksa paste or other Thai curry paste
(3)1 large can coconut cream (1 1/2 cups)
(4)2 cups mixed chopped vegetables (see note above)handful fresh basil leaves

Place noodles in a heatproof bowl and cover with boiling water. Allow to stand for 1 minute then massage to loosen into individual strands and drain. Meanwhile heat 2 tablespoons of peanut or other vegetable oil in a large saucepan over high heat. Add curry paste and stir fry for 30 seconds. Quickly add coconut cream and 2 cups boiling water. Bring to the boil and add vegetables. Simmer for 2 minutes or until the vegetables are cooked to your liking. To serve, divide noodles between 3 bowls. Pour over soup and vegetables and top with basil leaves

Zucchini (Courgette) Soup

The fastest way to grate zucchini is using a food processor. If you don't have one you could get some exercise and grate with a hand grater. Or just cut the zucchini into small chunks - they'll take a little longer to cook. To the herbs, add some freshness at the end but the soup will be lovely without it.

(1) 2 cloves garlic, finely sliced
(2) 4 medium zucchini, grated
(3) 2 cups tomato cassata
(4) 1/2 bunch basil or flat leaf parsley,
leaves picked parmesan cheese, to serve

Heat 2 tablespoons olive oil in a large saucepan and cook garlic over a high heat for 30 seconds or until just starting to brown. Add zucchini and cook stirring for a couple of minutes. Add cassata and 2 cups water and bring to the boil. Simmer for 7-8 minutes or until zucchini is tender. Taste and season and toss through herbs. Serve with cheese grated on the top.

Pea & Pasta Soup with Bacon

This is my take on the classic ham and pea soup. Frozen peas are a life saver when you're in the mood for something green and the larder is empty. Peas are one of those vegetables that start to lose their natural sweetness and flavour as soon as they are picked so unless you have access to peas straight from the plant, frozen will generally taste better. You can use bacon instead of ham and serve it in chunks on top but you could skip the bacon and use vegetable stock if you wanted a vegetarian soup.

(1) 4 rashers bacon
(2) 4 cups chicken stock
(3) 1/2 packet frozen peas (250g or 1/2lb)
(4) 200g or 7oz macaroni or other small

pasta

(5)1/2 bunch chives, chopped, optional

Cook bacon under a broiler or overhead grill until brown and crispy. Meanwhile bring the stock to the boil in a large saucepan. Add peas and pasta and boil for about 8 minutes or until the pasta is cooked. Stir through chives, if using. Taste and season as you serve soup topped with bacon pieces.

CHAPTER FIVE: SALADS AND VEGETABLES

I vary my ratios of oil to vinegar etc all the time. The recipes below should be taken as a guide only. Unless otherwise indicated they should make enough to dress a bag of prewashed leaves. But again it's all up to you. Caramelised red wine vinegar and wholegrain mustard is a favourite dressing at the moment, especially for a salad to accompany a big fry-up for brunch. If you can't find any, regular red wine vinegar with a teaspoon of honey makes a good substitute.

(1) tablespoon caramelised red wine vinegar
(2) 1 tablespoon wholegrain mustard
(3) 3 – 4 tablespoons extra virgin olive oil
(4) 2. aged balsamic & olive oil dressing
An oldie but a goodie. I love the sweetness of balsamic that is so well combined with the vinegar during the aging process that it seems to be almost savoury.

Classic to Dress Peppery Wild Rocket

(1) 2 tablespoon aged balsamic vinegar
(2) 4 tablespoons extra virgin olive oil

(3)3 tarragon vinegar & Dijon mustard dressing

Tarragon vinegar, tempers the flavour of fresh tarragon and gives an interesting twist. To make your own, just shove 1/2 bunch tarragon in a bottle of white wine vinegar and allow it to sit for a few weeks. It will keep for ages. This dressing is also lovely with a regular white wine or Champagne vinegar.

(1)1 tablespoon tarragon vinegar

(2)1 tablespoon Dijon mustard

(3)4 tablespoons extra virgin olive oil

Broccoli with Chickpeas & Tahini Sauce

This is broccoli at its best and it is crunchy and fresh in some spots, caramelised and complex in others. It seems like so much more than, well, just broccoli. Tahini is a paste of ground sesame seeds and is available from most health food stores. Natural yoghurt and lemon juice, without the water make a good substitute.

(1)1 head broccoli, chopped into bite sized mini-trees

(2)1 can chickpeas (14oz / 400g), drained

(3) 2 tablespoons tahini
(4) 3 tablespoons lemon juice
Preheat a large frying pan on the hottest heat. Add 2 tablespoon olive oil to pan. When it starts to smoke add the broccoli and cover with a lid or an oven tray – it's critical to seal it so the broccoli fries from the bottom but steams at the top. After 2 minutes, remove the lid and stir. Return lid and cook for a further 2 minutes. Add the chickpeas and stir. Cover and cook for another minute. Test a piece of broccoli – if it's tender, remove from the heat. If not, cover and cook for another few minutes. Meanwhile, combine tahini and lemon juice with 2 tablespoons water and stir until you have a smooth sauce. Serve broccoli and chickpeas with tahini sauce drizzled over the top.

Wilted Green with Parmesan

My favourite greens for this dish are either kale or Cavalo nero (also known as Tusan cabbage) but it's also lovely with plain old spinach or silver beet. It is one of the all time favourite single gal meals. It's also surprisingly versatile.

The cheese can be substituted with all manner of things. Sometimes I poach an egg, or just toast some pine nuts to sprinkle on top. It can also be a great way to use up leftover ragu or even risotto.

(1) 1-2 cloves garlic, peeled & finely sliced
(2) 1 bunch or about 4 large handfuls Cavalo Nero (or other greens – see note above)
(3) 1/2 lemon
(4) 1 handful grated parmesan cheese

Heat 2 tablespoon olive oil in a large frying pan or saucepan over a medium high heat. Add garlic and cook until it just starts to brown. Add greens and stir fry until just wilted. Remove from the heat. Squeeze through a little lemon juice. Taste and season as you serve on a warm plate with parmesan sprinkled over and extra lemon on the side.

Field Mushrooms with Feta & Olive Dressing

This is a great thing to serve vegetarian guests who will be so excited that you've gone beyond the standard veggie lasagne or risotto. The dressing also tastes great with lamb chops so you could cook up a few if you need to keep any carnivores placated. Serve with some crusty bread or mashed potato to soak up the mushroom dressing juices and a simple green salad.

(1) 4 large field mushrooms
(2) 3 tablespoons red wine vinegar
(3) 1 tablespoon Dijon mustard
(4) 200g (3 1/2oz) marinated feta handful small olives

Heat a large frying pan on the highest heat. Add a few tablespoons olive oil and add the mushies. Cover and cook for about 4 minutes. Turn and cook for another 4 minutes or until mushrooms are soft. Meanwhile, mix vinegar and mustard with 4 tablespoons extra virgin olive oil. When mushies are cooked, turn stalk side up. Divide clumps of feta between the mushrooms and drizzle over feta and olives. Allow the dressing to warm through before serving.

Mushroom, Macaroni Tuna Dish

(1) 1 large onion
(2) 1 can mushroom or celery soup
(3) Pinch mixed herbs ½ cup grated cheese
(4) Grated lemon rind
(5) 1 can tuna
(6) 1 cup cooked macaroni or rice
(7) ½ cup creamy milk
(8) 2 chopped gherkins

Fry onion. Add soup, milk and half cheese. Add tuna and gherkins – heat; add herbs, rind, and macaroni. Heat (if in a casserole dish top with cheese and heat under griller).

Macaroni Cheese

(1) 1 finely chopped onion
(2) ¼ teaspoon dry mustard
(3) 2 cups milk
(4) 1 tablespoon sherry
(5) 2 tablespoon plain flour
(6) salt

(7) pepper cayenne
(8) 1 egg
(9) 1 ½ cups shredded cheese
(10) 2 oz margarine
(11) ½ lb uncooked macaroni

Cook macaroni until tender and drain. Melt margarine and fry onions until soft but not browned.
Add flour and seasonings; gradually add milk and sherry stirring well until boiling. Pour into casserole and sprinkle with cheese and bake 20-30 minutes.ith corn flour if need to. Just before serving, add some to make a richer sauce.

Chicken or Veal Scaloppini

Cut chicken or veal into small bits (hammer if want) and put into plastic bag to coat with flour mixture of plain flour, oregano, salt, pepper and ground coriander. Fry coated meat in butter or oil in fry pan. Add chopped shallots and garlic. Add sauce of: tomato paste, sherry, chicken stock Powder, ½ cup water and parmesan cheese. Pour over meat and simmer till thickens. Add squeeze lemon juice at serving.

(1) Apricot Chicken
(2) Chicken breasts
(3) Apricot nectar can
(4) French onion soup (dried packet Cut full breasts in half. Brown floured chicken fillets, or places them in casserole without even browning them. Add nectar and packet soup and cover with foil or lid. Bake in moderate oven 45 minutes or till tender. (Or 15-20 mins in microwave).Quantities depend on number of breasts. If they are three to four3-4 breasts use medium can nectar and full packet of soup. You can thicken the sauce later.

(1) Chicken In Peanut Sauce
(2) Chicken thigh or breast
(3) 1 onion finely chopped
(4) 1 clove crushed garlic
(5) 30 g butter
(6) 1/3 cup peanut butter
(7) ½ cup chicken stock
(8) ¼ cup honey

(9)2 teaspoons grainy mustard
(10)1 teaspoon curry powder pinch cardamom
(11)dash Tabasco sauce (optional)

Fry onion and garlic, add chicken (sliced thin) and cook, add other ingredients.

Chicken with Onion Sauce

(1)1kg chicken drumsticks
(2)2 tablespoons oil
(3)60g butter
(4)1 onion
(5)400g can peeled tomatoes
(6)Packet dried French onion soup
(7)1 tablespoon soy sauce
(9)1 cup water
(10)3 teaspoons corn flour
(11)1 tablespoon water extra

Heat oil and half butter in pan, add drumsticks and brown all over. Remove.

Drain fat from pan, add remaining butter, peeled and sliced onion and cook till tender. Add mashed tomatoes that have not been drained of water, soup mix, soy sauce and water and cook till tender. Arrange chicken in ovenproof dish, pour sauce over and bake in moderate oven 45 minutes. Remove chicken to plates, pour sauce into pan and thicken with corn flour and water. Pour sauce over chicken.

CHAPTER SIX: MEAT BALLS WITH SWEET AND SOUR SAUCE

(1) 1 onion
(2) 1 small green pepper
(3) ½ clove garlic
(4) 1 stick celery
(5) 1 cup water
(6) ½ cup chopped sultanas or raisins
(7) 1 tablespoon vinegar
(8) 1 tablespoon chutney
(9) ½ teaspoon sugar
(10) salt, pepper
(11) 1 lb mince meat
(12) 2 chopped shallots
(13) 1 egg
(14) little milk if needed

Into saucepan place chopped onion, pepper, garlic and celery, add water, raisins, vinegar, chutney, sugar, salt and pepper. Bring to boil while preparing meat balls. Mix mince, shallots, egg and milk if needed. Shape into balls, brown in oil and drop into sauce. Simmer gently until meat cooked, 20 – 25 minutes.

Left over Meat

(1) 1 ½ cups cubed boiled potatoes
(2) 1 cup chopped cooked onions
(3) 1 ½ cups leftover cooked meat
(4) 1 tin cream of mushroom soup or celery soup
(5) salt, pepper
(6) any leftover veggies
(7) herbs

Fill greased casserole with layers of ingredients. Add soup. Cover and bake ½ hour in moderate oven.
(1) Quick Chilli Con Carne
(2) mince steak
(3) tin whole or crushed tomatoes
(4) chilli powder
(5) tin red kidney beans
(6) 1 tablespoon brown sugar (because of

tomatoes)
(7)60salt, pepper

Brown meat in little oil, add chilli powder and then other ingredients. Simmer ¾ hour.

Mince

Put meat in a little oil and add any finely chopped up veggies, include onions, salt, pepper and some flavouring like soy sauce or tomato sauce or tin tomato and some water to simmer for ¾ hour and thicken at end with corn flour mixed in a little cold water.

Veal Goulash

(1)Diced veal
(2)2 tablespoon plain flour
(3)2 teaspoon paprika
(4)salt, pepper
(5)1 teaspoon brown sugar
(6)Little oil
(7)2 large onions chopped

(8) 2 carrots diced
(9) 1 cup celery chopped
(10) 1 green pepper chopped

1 1/2 cups stock OR can add can drained pineapple pieces, tablespoon vinegar or 3/4 cup pineapple juice, 2 tablespoon soy sauce, 4 tablespoon sugar and corn flour for sweet/sour sauce. Coat the veal with flour, paprika, sugar, salt and pepper in a bag. Heat oil and fry meat till browned. Remove. Brown onions and sauté rest of veggies. Replace meat. Add stock. Cover and simmer gently 11/2 hours, or put in casserole in oven for 1 1/2 hrs. Thicken sauce if necessary with corn flour. Serve with rice.

Meat Loaf

(1) 750g mince
(2) 1/2 cup finely chopped onion
(3) 1 cup soft breadcrumbs
(4) 2 tablespoon chopped parsley

(5) 1 tablespoon Worstershire sauce
(6) 1 tablespoon tomato sauce
(7) 1 tablespoon mustard
(8) 1 egg
(9) 2/3 cup tinned carnation milk (not skim)
(10) 1/4 cup tomato sauce
(11) 1 tablespoon brown sugar
(12) 1/2 teaspoon dry mustard

Mix all meat ingredients in bowl and press into greased loaf tin. Bake in moderate oven 180C for 15 minutes. Gently remove loaf tin and brush with glaze. Return to oven for further 45 minutes at same temperature and serve hot or cold.

Hot Tuna Fritters

(1) 450g tin tuna
(2) 3 tablespoons flour
(3) 1 tablespoon baking powder
(4) 3 tablespoon milk
(5) 1 teaspoon chopped parsley
(6) 1 teaspoon lemon juice
(7) salt, pepper
(8) 2 eggs

Remove bones from fish – place it in a basin and break up, add milk and flour, baking powder, seasonings and beaten egg yolks. Whip egg whites stiffly and fold in lightly. Drop dessertspoons of mixture in hot oil and fry till golden.

Chicken in Onion Sauce

Put leftover cooked chicken into the following sauce and heat through. Sauté 1 chopped onion. Add:

(1) 1 400g can tomatoes
(2) 41g packet of dry French Onion soup mix
(3) 1 tablespoon soy sauce
(4) 1 cup water or chicken stock
(5) 3 teaspoons corn flour, to thicken.

Chicken Cacciatore

(1)dash oil(2)1 onion sliced
(2)1 tablespoon crushed garlic
(3)200g button mushrooms
(4)6 chicken thigh portions, boneless, skin removed
(6)½ cup white wine or water
(7)1 X 420g can condensed tomato soup
(8)Sprig fresh thyme

Heat oil in pan, and fry the onion, garlic and mushrooms for two minutes. Add chicken thighs and brown. Pour in wine or water and soup. Add thyme. Bring to boil, simmer covered for 30-35 minutes, until chicken tender. Serve with rice and green beans.

(1)Spanish Sauce:
(2)2 tablespoons margarine
(3)½ cup thinly sliced celery
(4)1 medium onion sliced
(5)1 small clove garlic chopped
(6)1 450g tin mashed tomatoes
(7)4 teaspoons sugar
(8) Salt, pepper

Melt margarine and sauté onion and celery, add all other ingredients and simmer 10 minutes.

Roast Lamb

Wipe leg of lamb with damp cloth and combine

(1) 1 dessertspoon salt
(2) 1 clove garlic chopped or crushed garlic or powder
(3) 1 level teaspoon dry mustard

Rub over the meat.

Place leg in baking dish with a little fat. Bake 1 – 1½ hours (depending on size of leg) at 180C. Remove some fat but leave a little in pan. Add– 1 cup strong black coffee, 1 teaspoon sugar and 1 dessertspoon cream. Baste the leg with this and bake 1 further hour. May have to add a little water if liquid reduces too much. Thicken sauce with flour and water, and serve at table in sauce jug.

(1) Lamb Chops In Orange Sauce
(2) 6 lamb chops (leg or chump)
(3) Flour seasoned with salt and pepper
(4) 1 cup orange juice
(5) Orange rind grated or 1 dessertspoon

orange marmalade
(6)¼ teaspoon nutmeg
(7)1 dessertspoon white vinegar
(8)2 onions
(9)1 potato per person

Dip chops in seasoned flour and fry till brown. Remove from pan. Add onions and potatoes and brown in pan. Place veggies in bottom of casserole and place chops on top. Combine rest of ingredients and pour over chops. Cover with foil and cook 1 hour in moderate oven. Serve with peas or salad.

Marinade for Barbeque Meat

Combine and shake well:
(1)Oil
(2)Vinegar or lemon juice
(3)Chopped onion
(4)Crushed garlic
(5)Salt, pepper, dry mustard

Soak meat overnight (at least 4-6 hours) turning several times.

For lamb add 1 teaspoon curry powder. For beef add ½ teaspoon oregano and 2 tablespoon Worstershire sauce. Cook meat on hot barbeque and brush over with marinade during cooking. Put all tough things in food processor with cutting blade, pinch salt and pepper, blend; add coriander seeds, lime juice and herbs, and 2 tablespoons oil. Blend/chop up.

Chicken curry:

Cut up skinless breast in big slices. Marinate 20min – 2 hrs in 1-2 tablespoons of above green paste. Heat oil and cook chicken to sear 2-3 minutes. Add paste and cook 30 seconds. Add coconut milk (can), stir and simmer 12-13 min until tender. Ad garnish of coriander leaves, coconut slices or nuts if wish.

Beef Curry In Sweet Peanut Sauce(1)500g beef cut into strips (or chicken or pork)
(2)3 tablespoons red curry paste
(3)1 can of coconut cream
(4)3 tablespoons brown sugar
(5)2 tablespoon fish sauce
(6)1/3 cup roasted ground peanuts
(7)1 tablespoon oil Heat oil, add curry paste for 1 minute. Add meat and stir fry for 2-3 minutes. Add coconut cream and

rest of ingredients. Simmer 15 minutes, stirring occasionally. Serve with rice.

Eggs in Celery Sauce

(1)3 cups hot boiled rice
(2)1 tablespoon chopped parsley
(3)5 hard boiled eggs
(4)salt, pepper
(5)paprika
(6)1 X 300g can cream of celery soup
(7)1/3 cup evaporated milk (or plain milk)
(8)½ cup grated cheese
(9)fine dry breadcrumbs
(10)grated Parmesan cheese

Put hot rice in shallow ovenproof dish, mix n parsley, top with eggs cut in halves lengthwise. Sprinkle over salt, pepper and paprika. Heat together soup, milk and grated cheese, stirring constantly. Pour over eggs, top with light dusting of crumbs mixed with some grated Parmesan cheese. Bake in moderately hot oven until heated through.

Eggs In Curry Cream(1)1 medium tomato peeled and chopped1 (2)clove garlic crushed
(3)1½ teaspoon curry powder

(4) ¾ cup sour cream
(5) 1/3 cup mayonnaise
(6) 3 cups hot boiled rice
(7) 2 teaspoons snipped chives
(8) French dressing
(9) 6 hard boiled eggs
Few blanched almonds split in halves
Fry tomato and garlic gently in little butter for a minute or two. Add curry powder and stir over low heat for 2-3 minutes, drain, put aside till cold. Push tomato mixture through sieve, stir into sour cream with mayonnaise and chill. Mix together rice and chives and moisten with French dressing, toss and chill. Fry almond halves in little oil till browned. Cut eggs in half lengthwise, put rice on serving platter, top with egg halves and coat with curry cream. Scatter over the almonds.

Fried Tempura

Dipping sauce:
Rice wine vinegar; add sugar and stir till clear and taste Ok (tang off). Add chopped coriander, chilli, garlic, salt and pepper. Stir well and taste. Cut up variety of veggies; remember thin slices for veggies

like sweet potato so can cook in oil 2-3 minutes.

Batter (made just before cook) :(1)1 cup corn flour

(2)2 cups plain flour

(3) Ice cold water or cold soda water

Stir in water with fork so still a bit lumpy and like thickened cream. Put in veggies and coat. Fry in hot oil 220oC (sunflower oil), Turn over, remove when crisp and drain on paper. Add salt. Serve with dipping sauce.

Savoury Impossible Pie

(1)3 eggs

(2)½ cup plain flour salt, pepper

(3)1 cup milk 60g melted margarine and add any of following – chopped onion, chopped bacon, celery, carrot, mushroom tomato, salmon, parsley, etc.

Mix all ingredients with fork. Pour into greased pie plate. Top with 1 cup grated cheese and bake at 180oC for ¾ hour till firm.

Spaghetti

Put mince (can add chopped onion if want) in glass bowl with lid on and cook on HIGH

4 minutes. Get out and break up meat with tongs or fork (as it tends to stick together), and drain off some of the fat/liquid (whilst running hot water down sink so fat doesn't clog pipes).Add the bottle of sauce, and frozen peas and/or corn to meat, mix.

Cook on high again for 4 – 6 minutes then boil water (1/2 full saucepan) on stovetop. When boiling, add spaghetti noodles and turn heat down to boil for about 10 minutes or until tender.

Part 2

Introduction

Congratulations on downloading *The Mediterranean Diet: Say Hello to Healthy Eating and Goodbye to Aging* and thank you for doing so.

The following chapters will discuss how to follow the plan and the ways it will most benefit your health. By following the Mediterranean diet plan, you will be consuming an abundance of vegetables, fruits, olive oil, legumes, and whole grains. The diet features lean choices of protein including poultry and fish instead of red meats which contain more saturated fat. You can also consume red wine moderately.

Each of the recipes has been planned specifically for the Mediterranean diet to ensure you are receiving the right balance of each of the essential nutrients. Some of the recipes may be listed in grams, and you will need to use a conversion chart.

When you see one, simply use the chart to convert to the desired measurement. You will notice throughout the readings the recipes will call for 'divided.' Essentially, this means you will be using the ingredient in more than one place in the recipe. You may also notice some abbreviations for a change of pace including:

- Tablespoon = T. or Tbsp.
- Teaspoon = t. or tsp.

There are plenty of books on this subject on the market, thanks again for choosing this one! Every effort was made to ensure it is full of as much useful information as possible; please enjoy!

Chapter 1: What is the Mediterranean Diet?

Origins of the Mediterranean Diet

Traditional foods are included from the 1960s from Greece and Crete, Southern Italy as the baseline for many of the menu plans. American researchers began to observe how these individuals had remained healthy in comparison to the people in the United States.

The first to associate with the Mediterranean diet was *The Seven Countries Study* which began in 1957 and has lasted for decades. The study involved Yugoslavia, Finland, the Netherlands, Japan, Greece, Italy, and the United States. The initial enrollment involved 12,000 healthy middle-aged men. Ancel Keys, the main investigator, discovered the seven countries had the lowest cardiovascular disease rates, apparently because of the diet planning of those areas.

Epidemiologic studies have indicated that individuals that consume a more typical 'Western' diet which is rich in dairy products, red meat, as well as salt and artificially sweetened foods will consume less of the legumes, fish, veggies, whole grains, and fruits provided in the Mediterranean Diet.

Many of the standard American diets are focused on fried or fast foods, refined carbohydrates, and many others which contain high levels of saturated or trans fats, as well as sodium. These plans lead to deficiencies in vitamins, minerals, and fiber.

Basics of the Mediterranean Diet Plan

The basis of the diet calls for plant foods which moderately low in animal foodstuffs. On the other hand, it is advised to eat seafood or fish for at least two days of the week. You will want to consume plenty of water, and as previously mentioned one glass of red wine daily is admissible. Coffee and tea are okay, but you should avoid sweeteners.

What to Eat:
- *Healthy Fats*: Olives, extra-virgin olive oil, avocado oil, and avocados
- *Dairy*: Greek yogurt, cheese, yogurt
- *Eggs*: Duck, chicken, quail
- *Poultry*: Turkey, duck, chicken
- *Whole Grains*: Brown rice, whole oats, barley, rye, whole wheat, buckwheat, corn, whole grain pasta, and whole grain bread, etc.
- *Spices and Herbs*: Cinnamon, garlic, mint, basil, sage, rosemary, pepper, nutmeg, etc.
- *Breads*
- *Seafood and Fish*: Tuna, salmon, trout, sardines, shrimp mackerel, oysters, shrimp, crab, clams, mussels, etc.
- *Vegetables*: Kale, broccoli, tomatoes, carrots, cauliflower, spinach, onions, cucumbers, Brussels sprouts

- *Tubers*: Sweet potatoes, potatoes, yams, turnips, etc.
- *Legumes*: Lentils, peas, beans, chickpeas, peanuts, pulses, etc.
- *Seeds and Nuts*: Macadamia nuts, cashews, almonds, walnuts, pumpkin seeds, hazelnuts, sunflower seeds, etc.
- *Fruits:* Dates, grapes, strawberries, oranges, apples, bananas, pears, peaches, melons, etc.

Note: Many of the Mediterranean Diet recipes call for olive oil; you will use the extra virgin type if it is not specified.

What to Eat in Moderation:
- *Eggs*
- *Poultry*
- *Yogurt*
- *Cheese*

Rarely Eat: *Red Meat*

Avoid These Foods:

- *Added Sugars*: Ice cream, candy, soda, table sugar
- *Sugar-Sweetened Beverages:* Avoid juices high in sugar
- *Refined Grains*: Pasta made with refined wheat, white bread
- *Trans fats*: Margarine and other processed foods
- *Processed Meat*: Hot dogs, processed sausages, etc.
- *Refined Oils:* Canola, cottonseed, soybean, and others
- *Higher Processed Foods:* Any foods marked 'diet,' 'low-fat,' or factory produced

Benefits of the Plan

- *Improved Weight Loss*: Individuals on the Mediterranean diet plan lost over three times more weight than those on other plans as stated by a New England Journal of Medicine.
- *Prevent Heart Attacks*: The reduced level of oxidized low-density

lipoprotein (LDL) cholesterol is evident with the plan.
- *Helps Prevent Strokes and Alzheimer's disease:* The reduction of blood sugar levels and general blood vessel health is improved.
- *Type 2 Diabetes*: Better control of sugar levels/blood glucose
- *Premature Death*: Over 1.5 million healthy adults have been associated with living a fuller life on the diet plan. That calculates to a 20% reduced risk of death rate at any age.
- *Improved Moods*: Over 15,000 individuals were studied in Spain and found the amounts of omega-3 fatty acids contributed to a lower risk of developing depression.
- *Keeps You Agile*: Muscle weakness and other frailty signs are reduced up to 70 percent.

You probably wonder how all of this is possible with the high fat in the diet. You are less likely to be hungry with the protein, fiber, and healthy fats entering your body. The veggies will make up the volume in the meals. These types of foods will not cause a spike in blood sugar, resulting in hunger in an hour or so. You can make it through the day without all of the extra snacks.

Essential Nutrients

Tips of How to Reap the Benefits

Adapting to a strict Mediterranean diet plan is best described by taking advantage of the methods used in a food pyramid of sorts. The following lists will provide essential information of how to balance the plan.

Monthly Goals: Four servings of red meat

Weekly Goals:
Fish: Five to six servings
Poultry: Four servings
Nuts, olives, pulses: Three to four servings
Eggs: Three servings

Potatoes: Three servings
Sweets: Three servings

Daily Goals:
Olive Oil: The main added lipid
Dairy Products: Two servings
Fruit: Three servings
Veggies: Six servings
Non-refined cereals and Similar Products: Eight Servings: This group includes brown rice, as well as whole grain pasta and bread.

Add some physical activity to the combination and drink plenty of water. Replace some of your salt intake with herbs such as thyme, basil, and oregano.

Chapter 2: Breakfast Recipes

Breakfast Couscous

This dish can be used for dinner with a bit of a twist, but this one has dried fruit and brown sugar which is ideal for four breakfast servings.

Ingredients
1 cup uncooked whole-wheat couscous
3 cups low-fat 1% milk
½ cup dried currants
1 (2-inch) cinnamon stick
½ cup dried apricots
¼ teaspoon salt
6 teaspoons (divided) dark brown sugar
4 teaspoons (divided) melted butter

Preparation
1) Using a medium-hi on the stovetop; place a large saucepan and add the cinnamon stick and milk. Heat it until you see bubble formations along the edges. (Don't boil.)

2) Take the pan off the burner and blend in the apricots, couscous, salt, currants, and 4 teaspoons of the brown sugar.

3) Place a lid on the pan and let it rest for 15 minutes.

4) Take the top off and throw away the cinnamon stick.

Serve it evenly in four bowls and garnish with ½ teaspoon of brown sugar, and a teaspoon of melted butter.

Banana Nut Oatmeal

Ingredients
2 tablespoons chopped walnuts
¼ cup quick cooking oats
1 teaspoon flax seeds
3 tablespoons honey
½ cup skim milk
1 peeled banana

Preparation

1) Mix everything together in a microwave-safe dish, except for the banana.
2) Cook two minutes on high.
3) With a fork, mash and stir in the banana.
Serve piping hot!

Mediterranean Breakfast Quinoa

Ingredients
1 cup quinoa
¼ cup chopped raw almonds
5 dried apricots
1 t. ground cinnamon
2 dried pitted dates
2 Tbsp. honey
1 t. sea salt
2 cups milk
1 t. vanilla extract

Preparation
1) Finely chop the dates and apricots.

2) Over medium heat, toast the almonds three to five minutes in a skillet. Set to the side.

3) Heat the quinoa, salt, and cinnamon using medium heat until warm. Pour in the milk.

4) When the mixture boils, reduce the heat, and place a lid on the saucepan, continue cooking slowly for approximately 15 minutes.

5) Pour in the honey, vanilla, apricots, dates, and ½ of the almonds.

6) Garnish with the rest of the almonds for a tasty treat.

Almond Biscotti

If you are searching for something to dip in your tea, cappuccino, or coffee; this is it!

Ingredients
1 pound flour
1 pound lightly toasted whole almonds
4 (+) 1 eggs
2 teaspoons vanilla

Zest of 2 lemons
1 teaspoon baking powder
½ pound sugar

Preparation
1) Preset the oven temperature to 350ºF.
2) Prepare a cookie sheet with parchment paper.
3) Slice the almonds into halves.
4) Mix four of the eggs and the remainder of ingredients in a large mixing bowl.
5) Process the dough into a 1 ½-inch thickness making three logs.
6) Place on the prepared baking sheet.
7) Beat and spread the last egg over the logs and bake for 30 minutes.
8) When it is ready, cut the logs into ½-inch wide slices.
9) Place it back in the oven at 300ºF for 25 more minutes.

Mediterranean Slices

85 g cheddar/grated or 125 g ball mozzarella cheese

375 g package ready-rolled puff pastry

140 g. container each:

- Frozen artichokes (3 wedges per serving)
- Sliced roasted peppers

4 tablespoons green pesto

Preparation

1) Set the oven temperature to approximately 395ºF/200ºC.

2) Unroll and cut the pastries into 4 rectangles (some may be pre-cut).

3) Spread 1 tablespoon of the pesto onto each of the four rectangles.

4) Add the artichokes and peppers.

5) Cook the slices for fifteen minutes in the preheated oven or just until the pastry begins turning brown.

6) Take the pan out and tear off the mozzarella ball into small bits, over the veggies.

7) Place it back into the oven and continue baking for another five to seven minutes.

8) Serve with a fresh green salad.

Avocado Egg Salad

Ingredients
Salt to taste
1 tbsp. lemon juice
2 hard-boiled eggs
3 green onions
1 avocado
3 tbsp. boiled corn
1 tbsp. olive oil
1 thinly chopped tomato

Preparation
1) Chop the green onions.
2) Blend the lemon juice and the finely chopped avocado in a large mixing container.
3) Mix the remainder of the components in the mixture (omit the tomato).
4) Serve with chopped tomatoes on bread slices.

Yields: 4

Mediterranean Eggs on Toast

Ingredients
2 slices whole wheat bread
4 eggs
6 black pitted olives
2 ounces sliced chorizo sausage
1 Tbsp. olive oil
2 Tbsp. milk
1 thinly sliced onion

Preparation
1) Whip/whisk the milk and eggs in a medium container, and set them to the side.
2) Using medium heat, pour the oil into a skillet; sauté the onion for four minutes.
3) Combine the sausage and continue cooking until crispy, approximately two to three minutes.
4) Toss in the olives and stir in the eggs. Cook for two minutes for a soft scrambled egg.
5) Toast the bread and add the egg on top with chives and pepper.

Yields: Two servings

Potato Hash and Chickpeas

Ingredients
1/2 cup onion
2 cups baby spinach
4 cups hash brown potatoes (frozen shredded)
1 tablespoon each:
- Curry powder
- Fresh minced ginger

¼ cup olive oil
1 Can (15-ounces) chickpeas
4 large eggs
½ teaspoon salt
1 cup zucchini

Preparation
1) Rinse the chickpeas thoroughly and chop the zucchini. Finely chop the onion and baby spinach.
2) Mix the onion, spinach, potatoes, salt, ginger, and curry powder in a large mixing bowl.

3) Using medium-hi, prepare a large skillet with the oil. Combine the potato mixture, and cook without stirring for about three to five minutes pressing it into a layer.

4) Lower the heat to medium-low. Blend in the zucchini and chickpeas, while breaking up the potatoes.

5) Press into an even layer once again.

6) In the center, carve out four 'wells,' while one at a time you place an egg into the 'well.'

7) Use a lid to cover the pan; continuing to cook for another four to five minutes for a soft yolk.

Chapter 3: Lunch Recipes

Two-Bean Greek Salad

Ingredients
4 ½ tsp. (divided)olive oil
1 (10-ounce) bag frozen lima beans or edamame
½ tsp. ground black pepper (divided)
3 tsp. fresh chopped oregano (divided)
2 tsp. Dijon mustard
2 tablespoons red wine vinegar
¾ pound string beans
1 cup halved grape tomatoes
3 ounces Ricotta Salata or Halloumi cheese
2 multigrain pitas
¼ cup pitted, halved Kalamata olives
1 cup grape tomatoes

Preparation
1) Slice the cheese into 4 pieces. Cut the tomatoes and pitas (horizontally) in half.
2) Blend the Dijon mustard, vinegar, 2 teaspoons olive oil, ¼ teaspoon of pepper,

and 2 ½ teaspoons oregano in a small serving dish. Place it to the side.

3) Put a steamer basket into a saucepan with several inches of water; cook the beans about three minutes covered. Remove them and put in a dish.

4) Put the string beans into the steamer and cook covered for about two minutes.

5) Combine the ingredients; add the olives and tomatoes. Toss the mixture to combine.

6) Serve on four plates, topping with the bean salad and cheese. Sprinkle the top of the finished product with the rest of the oil.

Yields: 4

Greek Avocado Salad

Ingredients

- 1 ½ pounds small tomatoes
- 2 cucumbers

- 1 ½ cups Kalamata (pitted & halved) olives
- ½ red onion
- ¼ cup flat leaf parsley
- 2 avocados
- 1 cup feta cheese in chunks
- 2 garlic cloves (peeled and minced)
- ½ cup red wine vinegar
- 2 teaspoons of sugar
- 1 teaspoon each:
- Black pepper
- Kosher salt
- 1 tablespoon oregano
- ½ cup olive oil

Preparation

1) Peel and cut the cucumbers into ½-inch slices/strips, quarter and steam the tomatoes, and chop the avocados into chunks. Thinly slice the onion. Chop the parsley.

2) Combine the onions, parsley, tomatoes, cucumbers, and olives in a large serving dish. Set the avocado in a dish to the side.

3) Combine the salt, pepper, sugar, garlic, oregano, vinegar, and oil in a canning jar or a similar container. Shake thoroughly.

4) Pour approximately 1 tablespoon of the dressing onto the avocado and coat it thoroughly. Use the rest on the cucumber mix and toss.

5) Place the avocado on the salad with the chunky feta, serve, and enjoy!

Garden Wraps

Ingredients

1 cup Greek yogurt

2 tomatoes

1 tablespoon chopped each:

- Cilantro
- Chives
- Fresh mint

½ teaspoon kosher salt

½ cup each:
- Cooked peas
- Sliced red onion

1 ½ cups each:
- Sliced cucumber
- Shredded carrots

4 sheets lavash

½ teaspoon kosher salt

Preparation

1) Cut the tomatoes in half and slice them thin.

2) Mix the salt, yogurt, and herbs in a small dish.

3) In another medium dish, mix the cucumber, carrots, cooked peas, and red onion.

4) Place 1 lavash sheet on countertop or platter, and add approximately ¼ of the mix of yogurt down the center, a layer of tomatoes, ¼ carrot mix, and fold/roll to one side of the flatbread.

5) Use several toothpicks to secure the ends.

6) Cut it in half and repeat with the remainder of the products.

Note: Lavash is a Mediterranean soft flatbread.

Serves: 4

Creamy Paninis

Ingredients

8 slices whole grain bread or ½-inch thickness

½ cup (divided) mayonnaise with olive oil

1/4 cup basil leaves (fresh is preferred)

7-ounces roasted red peppers (1 jar)

2 tablespoons chopped black olives

1 small thinly sliced zucchini

4 slices provolone cheese

Preparation

1) Finely chop the basil leaves.

2) In a small dish, mix the finely chopped olives with the mayonnaise.

3) Spread it on the slices of bread with the peppers, zucchini, and provolone. Top with the remainder of the slices.

4) Place mayonnaise on the outside of each sandwich.

5) On the stovetop using medium heat, place the sandwiches on a grill pan or skillet. Brown each of the sandwiches approximately four minutes.

6) What a treat with all of that melted cheese!

Yields: 4

Chicken

Chicken Souvlaki with Tzatziki

Ingredients
2 tablespoons lemon juice
14 ounces nonfat Greek yogurt
2 teaspoons fresh chopped oregano leaves
¼ cup white dry wine
¼ cup olive oil
½ teaspoon pepper (divided)
1 teaspoon kosher salt
2 pounds skinned, boneless chicken breasts

4 garlic cloves (2 minced & 2 crushed)
2 teaspoons distilled white vinegar
½ cup cucumber

Procedure

1) Cut the chicken into ½-inch cubes, and coarsely shred the cucumber.

2) Set the grill between 450º and 550º (hi).

3) Blend the wine, oil, chicken oregano, lemon juice, cloves, ¼ teaspoon of the pepper and the salt in a mixing bowl.

4) Use 8 metal skewers to place the chicken for cooking.

5) Grill for approximately 10 to 12 minutes.

6) Remove any excess moisture from the cucumbers with a towel, and put them into a medium dish. Mix in the yogurt, garlic, vinegar, and pepper with the cucumbers.

Serve with warm pita bread and the chicken.

Fish

Shrimp Pasta

Ingredients

- 1 pound medium shrimp
- 2 teaspoons olive oil
- 2 cups plum tomatoes
- 2 cloves garlic
- ¼ cup fresh basil
- 2 tablespoons drained capers
- 1/3 cup olives (Kalamata)
- 1/4 teaspoon black pepper
- ¼ cup (2-ounces) feta cheese
- 4 cups cooked angel hair pasta (uncooked 8-ounce package)
- Non-stick cooking spray

Preparation
1) Slice the basil thin, peel and devein the shrimp, chop the tomatoes, and mince the cloves. Pit and chop the olives. Prepare a skillet with cooking spray.

2) Cook the chosen pasta following the package instructions.

3) Add the garlic in a big pan with the oil using the med-hi setting. Sauté for 30 seconds.

4) Toss in the shrimp and continue to sauté for another minute.

5) Combine the basil and tomato—lower the heat—simmer for an additional three minutes.

6) Blend in the capers, olives, and pepper.

7) Place the shrimp and pasta in a salad dish to toss.

8) Sprinkle the top with the crumbled cheese.

Servings: 4

Scampi Greek-Style

Ingredients

- 1 pound medium shrimp
- 1 tsp. olive oil

- 6 ounces uncooked angel hair pasta
- 1 can diced tomatoes with garlic, basil, and oregano
    (14 1/2-ounces)
- 2 teaspoons garlic (bottled and minced)
- 1/8 tsp. each:
- Red pepper
- Ground black pepper
- ½ cup green bell pepper
- 6 Tbsp. (1 ½ ounces) feta cheese

Preparation

1) Peel and devein the shrimp. Chop the bell pepper and crumble the cheese. Use the liquid from the diced tomatoes—don't drain it.

2) Prepare the angel hair pasta according to the package instructions (omit the fat and salt). Drain and set aside to keep warm.

3) Use the med-high heat setting using a large pan to heat the oil.

4) Toss in the bell pepper and sauté for one minute. Add the tomatoes and garlic; continue cooking for another minute.

5) Combine the shrimp and black pepper—cover with a lid—and continue cooking for about three minutes.

6) Take the pan off the burner and toss in the red pepper.

7) Divide up the pasta and garnish with one cup of the shrimp goodies, and 1-½ tablespoons of the feta cheese.

Salmon with Slaw

In just 30 minutes you will be enjoying this mint slaw, rice, and salmon.

Ingredients
½ head (1 pound) cabbage
Pepper and Salt
1 cup brown basmati rice
½ cup fresh mint leaves
1 pound coarsely grated carrots
2 tablespoons grape-seed oil
2 teaspoons curry powder

4 (6-ounces) each salmon filets
¼ cup fresh lime juice (+) Wedges for serving

Procedure

1) Preheat the oven broiler and place a rack set within four inches from the heating coils.
2) Place aluminum foil over a baking sheet for the fish later.
3) Pour the rice into two cups of boiling water.
4) Flavor with pepper and salt—reduce the heat setting between low to medium and cook for thirty to thirty-five minutes.
5) Combine the carrots, cabbage, juice from the lime, mint, and oil or a dash of pepper and salt to taste in a large container. Toss the ingredients.
6) Approximately ten minutes from the time the rice will be ready put the salmon onto the prepared baking tin. Coat the salmon with the curry, pepper, and salt.
7) Broil six to eight minutes.
8) Fluff the rice with a fork.

What a meal of salmon, salad, and rice; perfect for lunch or brunch!

Note: There is no need to flip the salmon; it will cook thoroughly without the additional step.

Lamb

Lamb with Garlic & Rosemary

Ingredients

- 1 pound boneless leg of lamb (3/4-inch cubes)
- 4 (6-inch) whole wheat pitas
- 1 container (six-ounce) plain low-fat yogurt
- 1 t. minced garlic (bottled)
- ¼ (+) 1/8 t. black pepper
- 1/2 t. salt (divided)
- 1 T. fresh chopped rosemary
- 2 t. olive oil
- 1 T. lemon juice

- 1 ½ cups seeded cucumber (finely chopped)

Preparation

1) Use the med-hi setting to preheat the oil in a large pan.

2) Mix the rosemary, garlic, ¼ teaspoon each of salt and pepper, as well as the lamb as you toss it to coat.

3) Place the mixture into the pan and sauté four minutes.

4) Meanwhile, combine ¼ teaspoon salt, the lemon juice, cucumber, yogurt, and 1/8 tsp. of black pepper.

5) Place the lamb mix into the pitas and drizzle with the prepared sauce.

Cheesy Treats

Broad Bean and Feta Cheese Toasts

Ingredients
4 thin slices baguette (brown or white)
350 broad bean (frozen or fresh)
1 tablespoon olive oil

2 tablespoons mint leaves

50 g bag mixed leaf salad

1 teaspoon lemon juice

10 halved cherry tomatoes

100 g feta cheese/drained/vegetarian alternative

Preparation

1) Prepare a saucepan of boiling water, toss in the beans, returning to a boil, and continue cooking for around four minutes.

2) Run cold water over the beans using a colander. Drain.

3) Remove each of the beans from the skins, and set aside in a dish.

4) Mix the mint leaves and crumbled feta, toss well, and flavor with two tablespoons of the olive oil and a sprinkle of pepper. Mix again with the tomatoes and salad leaves with the lemon juice and balance of the oil.

5) Divide this into two serving dishes.

6) Toast the bread on both sides.

7) Spoon the cheese and bean mixture on the toast next to the salad.

Rigatoni with Asiago Cheese & Green Olive-Almond Pesto

Ingredients

- ½ cup fresh flat-leaf parsley leaves
- 6-ounces (1 ¼ cups) green olives
- 1 pound uncooked rigatoni
- 2 Tbsp. water
- 1/2 cup sliced toasted almonds
- 1 tsp. white wine vinegar
- ¼ tsp. freshly ground black pepper
- 1 large garlic clove
- 2 ounces (1/2 cup) grated Asiago cheese

Preparation

1) Prepare the rigatoni according to the package instructions (omit the fat and salt), and drain. Reserve 6 tablespoons of the liquid.

2) Use a food processor, and put the sliced almonds, olives, parsley leaves, garlic, and black pepper. Pulse the ingredients until they hold a coarsely chopped consistency (pulse three times).

3) Leave the processor ON, and add 1 teaspoon vinegar and 2 tablespoons of water; pulse until the ingredients are finely chopped.

4) Mix the olive combination and ¼ cup of the reserved liquids, as well as the pasta, in a large mixing dish; tossing well.

5) Only add enough of the remainder of the liquid to make the pasta maintain its moist consistency.

6) Sprinkle with the cheese and enjoy!

Serves: 6 (1 2/3 cups each serving)

Mediterranean Quinoa Salad

This is a great idea for a light lunch. If you need something on the side for dinner, this is also the answer to your dilemma.

Ingredients
1 cup uncooked quinoa
1/3 cup red wine vinegar
¼ cup olive oil
2 cups water
1 small diced red onion
1 diced red pepper
½ cup Kalamata olives
Juice of 1 lemon
½ cup chopped fresh cilantro
½ teaspoon black pepper
1 teaspoon salt
½ cup crumbled feta cheese
2 Roma tomatoes

Procedure
1) First, you will need to dice the tomatoes, onions, and peppers.
2) Over medium heat, prepare the water to boiling and add the quinoa. Lower the heat and continue to cook slowly for fifteen to twenty minutes. The water should be completely absorbed. Fluff and cool for five minutes.
3) Add the vinegar and oil—as the quinoa comes to room temperature.

4) Blend in the tomatoes, onion, olives, red peppers, cilantro, pepper, and salt.
5) Gently blend and add the feta cheese.
6) Chill in the refrigerator for about two hours, so the flavors can intertwine.
7) Before serving, spruce it up with a touch of lemon juice.

Broiled Feta with Olives & Roasted Peppers

Ingredients
1 each yellow and red pepper
1 Vidalia onion
8 ounces feta cheese
1 head garlic
1 tsp. olive oil
1 Tbsp. regular capers/8 caper berries
12 green olives or tsakistes (pitted)
8 anchovies
12 Kalamata olives (pitted)
Juice of 1 lemon
¼ cup each:
- Chives
- Mint

- Dill
- Fresh parsley

Preparation

1) Slice the peppers into halves, lengthwise. Separate the cloves and peel. Slice the onion into rounds.

2) Preheat the oven to 400ºF.

3) Using a baking sheet, put the garlic, onion, and peppers; brush them with some oil and bake for approximately twenty minutes.

4) Take from the oven, place the veggies on a covered dish or under some tight-fitting wrap.

5) Reset the broiler setting on the oven.

6) Use a baking sheet or casserole dish to crumble the feta. Broil until it bubbles—approximately two minutes.

7) Blend the remainder of the ingredients in a large mixing dish. Combine the onions, garlic, and peppers; tossing well.

8) Take the cheese from the broiler and spoon into the serving plates.

9) Garnish with the pepper mixture.

Complement the meal with some pita chips or pita bread.

Servings: 6

Brussels Sprouts With Honey Pomegranate and Apples

Ingredients
1 large Granny Smith apple
1 pound Brussels sprouts
1 diced medium onion
4 tablespoons oil
½ cup whole grain freekeh
¼ - 1/3 cup dried cranberries
2 tablespoons honey
¼ - 1/3 finely chopped parsley
Juice of ½ medium lemon
Arils of ½ large pomegranate
Black pepper
¼ teaspoon salt

Preparation

1) Preheat the oven to 400ºF. Use parchment paper to prepare a cookie sheet.

2) Peel, core, and dice the apple. Also, remove the outer leaves of the sprouts (peel) and cut in half if they are large.

3) Bring 1 ½ cups of water to boil in a small pan, and toss in ½ cup of freekeh.

4) Let the ingredients in the pan once again come to a boil, and lower the heat to simmer, covered for twenty to twenty-five minutes which will provide you with 1 ½ cups finished product. Take it from the burner and let it rest for five minutes. Drain out the rest of the water.

5) Combine 1/8 teaspoon salt and 2 tablespoons of oil with the sprouts and put them onto the baking sheet for approximately twenty minutes, flipping once after 15 minutes or until they are the desired consistency. Set the sprouts to the side.

6) Using the low-medium setting, use a large sauté pan with two tablespoons of oil, adding the onions for a few minutes. (Don't caramelize the onions.)

7) Combine the lemon juice and apple to the onions and sauté a few more minutes being careful not to let them get soft and mushy.

8) Toss in 1/8 teaspoon of salt, honey, and some pepper; continue to sauté for several minutes.

9) Combine the sprouts and freekeh to the pan and heat everything for several minutes to warm—not hot.

10) Remove from the burner and toss in the parsley, pomegranate seeds, cranberries, pepper, and salt.

11) Enjoy it at room temperature or warmed.

Notes: If you are not familiar with freekeh; it is a cereal food made from wheat that has been rubbed and roasted to enhance its flavor. It is also sometimes called farik and originates in the Mediterranean Basin.

You can prepare the freekeh and sprouts several days in advance if stored in an air-tight container.

Yields: 4 Servings

Chapter 4: Dinner Recipes

Easy Greek Casserole

Ingredients
Herbs such as basil, dill, & oregano to taste
1 bag baby spinach
1 tablespoon minced garlic
1 small finely chopped onion
1 tablespoon olive oil
1 ½ cups brown or wholegrain rice (quinoa is good)
1 can diced tomatoes or 1 pint grape tomatoes
1 cup sliced mushrooms
½ block firm tofu
2 beaten eggs
½ cup crumbled feta cheese
Sliced black olives

Preparations

1) Preheat the temperature of the oven to 375ºF.

2) Lightly grease an 'eight x eight' pan with cooking spray.

3) Drain and press the block of tofu.

4) Prepare the rice or other pasta as instructed on the package.

5) Preheat a skillet and pour in the oil.

6) Wash and squeeze dry the spinach.

7) Sauté the garlic and onion in the prepared pan until softened. Blend in the eggs, spinach, and other herbs—continue cooking until the spinach is wilted—usually for one or two more minutes.

8) Place the rice on the bottommost layer of the pan, and top with the spinach-rice mixture.

9) Combine the sliced olives and tomatoes in layers; cover with foil and continue cook in the oven for approximately twenty minutes.

10) Combine the feta and tofu until crumbly using a fork.

11) Take the casserole out of the oven and add the tofu-cheese topping. Place it back in the oven for another fifteen minutes.

It is time to when the toppings turn brown!

Stuffed Grape Leaves Casserole

Ingredients
1 large onion
30 fresh or jarred grape leaves
1 cup brown rice
2 Tbsp. olive oil
2 cups low-sodium vegetable or tomato juice
1 Cup each:
- Dried currants or raisins
- Fresh chopped mint
- Fresh chopped parsley
- Chopped hulled and unsalted pistachios

¼ cup lemon juice
Garnish: 1 sliced lemon
Brushing: More oil will be needed for brushing for this recipe

Preparation
1) Dice the onion in to fine bits.

2) Set the oven temperature at 350 F.

3) Grease a two-quart baking dish with oil.

4) Using the medium heat setting, preheat the oil in a big saucepan.

5) Prepare a large pot of boiling water. Place the leaves in the water two minutes; drain—set to the side.

6) Sauté the onion 7 to 10 minutes in the prepared pan; throw in the 2 ½ cups of water and rice; bringing the mixture to a boil.

7) Place a lid on the pan, lower the heat the med-low, and continue cooking for 30 to 40 minutes (the liquid will be absorbed).

8) Take from the burner, and blend in the parsley, pistachios, tomato juice, raisins, lemon juice, and mint. Flavor the mix with pepper and salt.

9) Place the leaves around the base and sides (drape them over the sides), putting 1/2 the rice mixture in the leaves. Add more leaves and use the remainder of the rice mix for a garnish.

10) Coat the baking dish with the rest of the leaves and seal with the edges of the grape leaves.

11) Brush with olive oil and bake 30 to 40 minutes.

12) The leaves will be dark, with the casserole looking dry and firm.

13) Dip a knife into cold water and cut into eight servings, removing them with a spatula.

14) Garnish with a drizzle of pomegranate molasses and lemon slices.

Yields: 8 servings

Chicken

Grilled Chicken with Quinoa Greek Salad

Ingredients

400 g chicken mini-fillets
225 g quinoa
1 red chili

1 ½ tablespoons olive oil
25 g butter
1 garlic clove
1 red onion
300 g tomato
1 red onion
Small bunch mint leaves
Handful black pitted Kalamata olives
Juice and zest from ½ lemon
100 g feta cheese

Preparation

1) Deseed and finely chop the red chili, roughly chop the tomatoes, and chop the mint leaves.

2) Prepare the quinoa according to the package instructions; rinse and drain completely.

3) Combine the garlic, butter, and chili into a paste.

4) Coat the chicken with 2 teaspoons olive oil.

5) Cook using a hot pan for 3 to 4 minutes per side.

6) Put on a dish and dot with spicy butter and set to the side.

7) Mix the tomatoes, olives, onion, mint, and feta in a medium bowl. Throw in the quinoa.

8) Blend in the lemon juice, zest, and the remainder of the oil.

9) Serve the fillets drizzled with the chicken juices.

Grilled Chicken and Grape Skewers

Ingredients

1/2 tsp. crushed red chili flakes
1 tablespoon each:
- Lemon juice
- Rosemary
- Oregano

¼ cup (+) 2 Tbsp. (divided) olive oil
1 pound chicken breast (no skin or bone)
2 minced garlic cloves
1 ¾ cups green seedless grapes
½ tsp. salt

1 tsp. lemon zest
12 skewers

Preparation

1) Clean the grapes and rinse them thoroughly.

2) Cut the chicken into ¾-inch cubes.

3) Blend the garlic, oil, chili flakes, oregano, rosemary, and lemon zest. Whip them together as the marinade.

4) Alternate the grapes and chicken onto the skewers.

5) Place them into a container to marinate from four to twenty-four hours.

6) Take the skewers from the container and let the oil roll away for a few minutes.

7) Drizzle with salt and grill three to five minutes per side.

8) Put them on a serving dish and splash some lemon juice and a bit of oil.

Servings: 4 entrees

Lemon-Zaatar-Grilled Chicken

Ingredients
4 (6 to 8-ounces each) chicken thighs
1 teaspoon lemon zest
1 lemon cut into 4 wedges
2 tablespoons lemon juice
8 green onions
1 teaspoon minced garlic
¼ teaspoon each pepper and salt

Procedure
1) Blend the zest, oil, lemon juice, zaatar, pepper, garlic, and salt in a big container. Put the thighs into the mix and fully cover the surfaces.
2) Use a medium grill temperature setting ranging between 350º to 450º. Place the chicken on the surface—skin side down—for five to eight minutes.
3) Flip the thighs and cook for approximately four additional minutes.
4) For the last few minutes, grill the onions and lemon wedges—flipping once.
Enjoy!

Note: The zaatar for this recipe can be located in the Middle Eastern section of most superstores.

Easy & Quick Gyros with Tzatziki Sauce

Ingredients
4 pitas
4 chicken breasts
½ red onion
1 red pepper
1 tablespoon Mediterranean seasoning/Italian seasoning
Optional: Crumbled feta cheese and lettuce

Tzatziki Sauce:
1/3 cup chopped dill (frozen or fresh)
4 tsp. minced garlic
1/8 tsp. black pepper
½ tsp. salt
2 cups plain Greek yogurt
1 ½ Tbsp. lemon juice
½ a cucumber

Preparation

1) To prepare the chicken, pound it to a ½-inch thickness for even cooking. Thinly slice the onion and peppers.

2) Puree each of the sauce components and place in the refrigerator. The flavors will combine as the mixture marinates.

3) Flavor the breasts with the seasoning and cook over medium heat in a large pan for about five to six minutes for each side. Slice them into strips.

4) Put the pitas together and garnish as you wish folder in a 'tunnel shape' or like a sandwich.

Note: You might need to use a food processor/blender for the puree. If you like a thicker sauce, remove as much liquid from the cucumbers before they are added to the pureed sauce.

Serves: 4

Chicken Kofte & Zucchini

Ingredients

¼ cup dry bread crumbs

½ cup store-bought tzatziki (divided)

5 Tbsp. fresh chopped mint (divided)

¼ cup grated onion

3/8 tsp. black pepper (divided)

1 tsp. ground cumin

1/8 tsp. ground red pepper

4 zucchini

5/8 tsp. kosher salt (divided)

1 pound ground chicken

4 tsp. olive oil (divided)

Procedure

1) Slice the zucchini lengthwise and halved.

2) Preheat the oven broiler to high. Use some cooking spray to coat a jelly-roll pan.

3) Blend the breadcrumbs, ¼ cup tzatziki, 3 tablespoons of the mint, onion, cumin, ¼ teaspoon black pepper, the red pepper, and ½ teaspoon salt in a container.

4) Blend in the ground chicken and mix thoroughly. Form the mixture into eight patties.

5) Use medium heat with 2 teaspoons of oil to cook the patties four minutes per side.

6) While to kofte is cooking, place the zucchini with the cut-side facing upwards in the jelly pan. Coat it with the remainder of the oil and drizzle it with the pepper and salt.

7) Broil about five minutes.

8) Garnish each of the four servings with 2 tablespoons of mint.

9) Serve the dish with the remainder of tzatziki.

Notes: In case you don't know, kofta is from the meatball family dishes found in Asian countries.

Lamb

Grilled Lamb Chops and Mint

Ingredients

½ cup chopped mint leaves (+) more for garnish

1/3 cup olive oil
Sea salt
¼ teaspoon red pepper flakes
2 smashed cloves garlic
2 1/3 pounds or 12 small rib lamb chops

Preparation
1) Set the grill to med-hi setting.
2) Blend the olive oil, red pepper flakes, salt, and mint in a mixing bowl.
3) Use the garlic to rub the chops.
4) Add a few tablespoons of the mint in a container to cover the lamb.
5) Grill the chops approximately three to four minutes on both sides or until charred.
6) Put the chops onto a serving dish and brush with the remainder of the mint oil mixture.
7) Garnish with some bits of mint.

Note: Medium rare consistency is when you push down on the center of the chop and it is somewhat firm.

Servings: 6

Turkey

Hummus Turkey Sliders

Ingredients

- 16 mini-pocket pitas
- 1 diced cucumber
- 2 Tbsp. red wine vinegar
- 4 Tbsp. olive oil
- 1 tsp. dried mint
- 2 to 3 sliced plum tomatoes
- 1/2 cup chopped fresh parsley
- 1 cup hummus (approximately 7-ounces)
- 2 tsp. ground coriander

Preparation
Place these in the fridge with a tight cover:

- Feta
- Cucumber
- Mint
- Vinegar
- Pinch each of pepper and salt
- 1 tablespoon oil

1) Blend ½ cup hummus, the turkey, coriander, and parsley in a mixing container.

2) Flavor with the pepper.

3) Prepare 16 small patties approximately ½-inch thick.

4) Use a large pan to heat the rest of the oil and cook each of the patties approximately two minutes for each side.

5) Combine the remainder of the hummus with a sprinkle of hot water in a mixing dish.

6) Place a portion of the hummus on the inner section of the pita.

7) Combine the turkey patty, tomato slice, and some of the cucumber mixture.

Notes: The pita is preferably whole wheat.

Beef

Beef Steaks Crusted in Cumin with Olive-Orange Relish

Ingredients
2 (3/4-inch) 8-ounce steaks
1 to 3 medium oranges
½ tsp. black pepper
1 tsp. salt
1 ½ - tsp. ground cumin
1/3 cup each:
- Red diced onion
- Kalamata olives (coarsely chopped)
- Chopped roasted red peppers

Preparation
1) Warm up a large skillet or grill pan using the medium heat setting.
2) Grate two teaspoons orange peel from the oranges and set the oranges to the side.

3) Peel—section—and chop 1- ½ cups oranges.

4) Mix the salt, cumin, and orange peel into a small dish. Save two teaspoons as seasoning for relish.

5) Combine the pepper to the seasoning and place on each of the steaks.

6) Put the steaks in the prepared skillet and cook from nine to twelve minutes—turning twice.

7) Blend the roasted peppers, oranges, onions, and reserved seasonings in a medium dish. Blend them well.

8) Serve with the relish.

Note: Beef shoulder steaks/ranch steaks are a good choice.

Yields: 4 servings

Kofte in a Hurry

This is a versatile recipe and can be made from beef, ground lamb or some of each. You can cook it on the grill on a stick or as described here on pita halves.

Ingredients

- ¼ cup fresh chopped mint
- 1 pound lean ground round meat
- 1/3 cup dry breadcrumbs
- ½ cup white onion – pre-chopped
- ½ tsp. salt
- 1 tsp. minced – bottled garlic
- 2 Tbsp. tomato paste
- 1/4 tsp. ground cinnamon
- ½ tsp. cumin
- 1/8 tsp. allspice
- ¼ tsp. ground red pepper
- 1 large egg white (slightly beaten)

¼ cup plain yogurt
2 plum tomatoes (8 - ¼-inch slices)
Cooking spray
4 (6-inch) split pitas

Preparation

1) Coat a jelly-roll pan with a small amount of oil or some cooking spray.

2) Preset the oven temperature to Broil.

3) Blend together the first set of ingredients (12 with the dots), and make 8 (2-inch) patties.

4) Put the patties in the pan and broil each side for four minutes.

5) Place the tomato, a patty, and top off each one with 1 1/2 teaspoons of yogurt in each of the pita halves.

Chickpea Patties

Ingredients

½ cup flat-leaf fresh parsley

1 can chickpeas (15.5-ounces)

¼ teaspoon cumin

1 garlic clove

1 whisked egg

½ teaspoon (divided) each:
- Kosher salt
- Black pepper

½ cup low-fat Greek-style yogurt

4 tablespoons (divided) all-purpose flour
2 tablespoons oil
8 cups mixed salad greens
3 tablespoons lemon juice
1 small red onion
1 cup grape tomatoes
Optional: Pita chips

Preparation
1) Preheat some oil in a skillet.
2) Rinse and drain the chickpeas. Chop the garlic clove, halve the tomatoes, and slice the red onion thin.
3) Use a food processor to pulse the first four ingredients (through the garlic clove), and add ¼ teaspoon each of the pepper and salt until the mixture is chopped coarsely and holds form.
4) Place the mixture in a bowl; blend the egg, and two tablespoons of the flour.
5) Make ½-inch patties.
6) Roll the patties in the remainder of the flour.
7) Use med-hi heat and place the patties into the prepared pan, and cook them for two to three minutes for each side.

8) Whip together the lemon juice, yogurt, and rest of the pepper, and salt.

9) Divide the onions, greens, tomatoes, and patties and sprinkle with about 2 tablespoons of the dressing over each of the salads.

10) Add pita chips on the side.

Yields: 4 servings 2 patties each

Seafood and Fish

Lemon Salmon and Lima Beans

Ingredients

- 4 (5-ounce) center-cut skinless salmon fillets
- 1-pound baby lima beans (frozen)
- ½ cup nonfat plain Greek yogurt
- 1 lemon
- ¾ teaspoons paprika
- 3 thinly sliced cloves garlic
- 1 ½ cups of water

- Pinch of red pepper flakes
- ¾ teaspoon dried oregano
- Black pepper
- Kosher salt
- 2 tablespoons fresh chopped parsley
- 2 teaspoons olive oil

Preparation

1) Preset the oven onto the broiler function.

2) Cover a cookie sheet with foil. Put 1 teaspoon of the oil in a medium saucepan and preheat.

3) For ½ of the lemon, slice it into 4 thin rounds; on the other grate the zest and set it to the side for later.

4) Combine some of the juice in a dish, add ¼ teaspoon of the paprika and the yogurt.

5) Place the garlic, oregano, and red pepper flakes in the pan and cook approximately two minutes.

6) Add the water, beans, and lemon zest; simmer for approximately 20 minutes.

Flavor the mixture with the pepper and salt if desired.

7) Take the pan from the burner and add 1 tablespoon of the paprika-yogurt mixture, parsley, and rest of the oil.

8) In the meantime, in a small dish, combine ½ teaspoon of the salt, ½ teaspoon of paprika, and pepper if desired. Add by drizzling over the salmon.

9) Place the salmon on the prepared pan and top each of the salmon fillets with a slice of lemon.

10) Broil for about six to eight minutes.

11) Enjoy the salmon with the lima beans and garnish with the paprika-yogurt mixture.

Servings: 4

Bass with Mushrooms and Spaghetti Squash

The sauce prepared with this delicious dish is a traditional Agrodolce sweet and sour sauce used by many Italian cuisine recipes.

Ingredients

- 4 (6-ounce) striped bass fillets
- 2 cups cherry tomatoes
- 12 ounces mixed mushrooms
- 5 Tbsp. olive oil (divided)
- Pinch of red pepper flakes
- 3 to 4 sprigs fresh rosemary
- 1 head garlic
- ¼ cup red wine vinegar
- 1 medium spaghetti squash
- 3 tablespoons sugar
- Fresh ground black pepper
- Kosher salt

Preparation
1) Prepare the temperature setting of the oven at 375ºF.
2) Use a small pan, and add three Tbsp. of olive oil using the low heat setting.
3) Prepare a baking sheet with foil.

4) Remove the pin bones from the bass. Cut the mushrooms into pieces if they are large. Peel the garlic and remove the seeds from the squash and cut it lengthwise.

5) *Prepare the sauce*: Add the whole garlic clove, rosemary, and pepper flakes to the prepared pan, stirring for about 8 minutes until the garlic is tender. (Save 1 tablespoon of the garlic oil.)

6) Add the sugar and vinegar and simmer using med-low heat for about five minutes until caramelized and syrupy.

7) Brush each side of the squash halves with the garlic oil and flavor with pepper and salt.

8) Put the squash in the baking dish (cut-side up), and roast approximately one hour.

9) Lower the heat to 200ºF.

10)Remove the flesh from the squash with a fork while you are holding it in your hand with a towel. Place the strands onto the baking dish. Flavor with pepper and salt, place foil over the tray and place in the warm oven for later.

11) Using med-high heat, add one tablespoon oil and the mushrooms; drizzle with a dash of salt, and stir about 10 minutes. Put on a serving platter.

12) Add the remainder of oil to the pan and simmer until the tomatoes are blistered. Combine 1 tablespoon of the sauce and a sprinkle of water. Cover and continue cooking for another five minutes. Place the mushrooms into the pan to warm.

13) Over the medium-high setting, place a saucepan with 1-inch of water. Flavor the fish with pepper and salt. Place a collapsible steamer or bamboo over the burner/water and steam for five to six minutes.

14) Take it from the burner and allow the mixture to rest for two to four minutes.

15) Serve with the fillet, mushrooms, squash, and tomatoes.

16) Garnish with a drizzle of sauce, and serve with the caramelized garlic and remainder of the sauce.

Notes: You can use a combination of chanterelle, shiitake, or oyster mushrooms.
Servings: 4

Mussels with Olives and Potatoes

Ingredients

- 2 1/4 pounds scrubbed mussels
- 1 medium sliced onion
- 2 large potatoes
- 2 Tbsp. olive oil
- 1/2 cup fresh parsley (roughly chopped)
- ½ tsp. paprika
- 1 ½ tsp. kosher salt
- 4 sliced cloves garlic

- 1 cup water

- 1 can diced tomatoes (14.5-ounce)
- A pinch each of:
    - Cayenne pepper
    - Allspice
- 2/3 cup halved and pitted green olives

Preparation

1) Preheat a Dutch oven/a large pot with the olive oil.

2) Cut the potatoes into 1-inch chunks.

3) Place the potatoes with ¼-inch of water using a microwave-safe container. Place some plastic wrap over the top and cook approximately 6 minutes until tender; drain them.

4) Combine the garlic and onion into the preheated pan and sauté for five to six minutes.

5) Toss in the paprika, potatoes, allspice, 1 ½ teaspoons of salt, and the cayenne into the mixture. Cook for approximately 2 to 3 minutes keeping the potatoes coated.

6) Pour in the water, and the tomatoes bringing it to a simmer. Place a lid on the pot and cook for around 10 minutes.

7) Combine the olives, parsley, and mussels into the pot, put the lid on, and cook for 4 to 5 more minutes.

Note: Throw away any mussels that do not open.

Seared Tuna Steaks

Ingredients
1/8 teaspoon black pepper
½ teaspoon ground coriander
½ teaspoon salt (divided)
4 (6-ounce) ¾-inches thick Yellow-fin tuna steaks
Cooking spray

Tomato Mixture:
½ tsp. minced garlic (bottled)
12 pitted chopped Kalamata olives
1 Tbsp. olive oil
1 Tbsp. drained capers

3 Tbsp. fresh chopped parsley
¼ cup green chopped onions
1 Tbsp. lemon juice
1 ½ cups seeded chopped tomatoes

Preparation
1) Use medium-hi heat, and place a large pan with the cooking spray added.
2) Drizzle the fish with the pepper, coriander, and ¼ teaspoon of salt and add to the pan.
3) Cook four minutes per side.
4) Blend the remainder of the ingredients.
5) Garnish the fish with the tomato mixture for a special taste treat.
Serves: 4

Side Dishes

Mushroom Kabobs

Ingredients
1 pound cremini mushrooms
2 tablespoons olive oil
Dash of black pepper

¼ cup balsamic vinegar
½ teaspoon each:
- Dried basil
- Dried oregano

Kosher salt

2 tablespoons freshly chopped parsley leaves

3 pressed garlic cloves

Preparation

1) Preset the oven temperature to 425ºF.

2) Cover a cookie sheet with a bit of oil.

3) Whip the oil, vinegar, oregano, garlic, and basil in a large container.

4) Combine with a dash salt or pepper, then, add the mushrooms.

5) Let the mixture rest for about ten to fifteen minutes.

6) Push the mushrooms onto skewers and place on the cooking sheet.

7) Roast approximately 15 to 20 minutes.

Sprinkle with parsley as a garnish.
Serves: 6

Mediterranean Potato Salad

Ingredients
300 g new potatoes
1 crushed garlic clove
1 teaspoon dried or fresh oregano
1 small onion
1 tablespoon olive oil
½ can (400 g) cherry tomatoes (more or less)
25 g sliced black olives
100 g roasted red pepper (from a jar and sliced)
Handful of torn basil leaves

Preparation
1) Using a small pan, combine the onion and the oil, and sauté for five to ten minutes.
2) Combine the oregano and garlic, continuing to cook for about one more minute.
3) Blend the peppers and tomatoes, flavor, and simmer for 10 minutes.

4) Put some salt into a pan and bring it to boiling. Put the potatoes in to cook for approximately 10 to 15 minutes.
5) Drain, mix with the sauce, and serve it warm.
6) Garnish with basil and olives for a tasty treat.

Roasted Peppers—Anchovies—and Tomatoes

Ingredients
1 (50 g) can anchovy in oil (drained)
4 red peppers
2 garlic cloves
8 small tomatoes
2 rosemary sprigs
2 tablespoons olive oil

Preparation
1) Cut the tomatoes and peppers in half and deseed the peppers. Thinly slice the garlic clove.
2) Preheat the oven to 320º F or 160º C.

3) Place the peppers on a large baking tin/dish and sprinkle with some of the anchovy oil. Turn the cut-side up.

4) Bake for approximately 40 minutes.

5) It should be soft but not to the point of collapsing.

6) Prepare the anchovies by slicing 8 of them lengthwise.

7) In each of the peppers, place the rosemary sprigs, 2 slices of anchovy, and 2 (1/2 pieces) of tomato. Sprinkle with the olive oil and bake about 30 minutes.

8) Serve at room temperature or when slightly warm.

Herbed Mashed Potatoes with Greek Yogurt

Ingredients
4 pounds yellow potatoes
1 cup Greek yogurt (whole milk)
¼ teaspoon pepper
2 teaspoons kosher salt (divided – more or less)
1/3 cup each chopped:

- Chives
- Dill
- Parsley

3 tablespoons softened butter (divided)
1 cup warm milk

Toppings:
2 tablespoons each chopped:
- Dill
- Chives
- parsley

Preparation

1) Yukon gold (thin-skinned) potatoes were used in this recipe; begin by peeling and cutting them into 1-inch chunks.

2) Place enough water and one tsp. of salt into a soup pot or similar pot to cover the potatoes.

3) Let the potatoes boil using the high heat setting. Lower to the medium setting, and boil about 15 minutes.

4) Turn off the burner, drain the potatoes, and place them back into the pot.

5) Combine 1/2 teaspoon salt, the yogurt, and 1/3 each of the dill, parsley, and chives. Set to the side.

6) Break up the hot potatoes with a potato masher.

7) Combine the 2 tablespoons of butter, milk, the pepper, and ½ teaspoon salt. Mash the potatoes until fluffy.

8) Blend the yogurt into the potatoes.

9) Add to the serving dish, and garnish with the butter that remains, with the chopped herbs.

Notes for Leftovers or Make them Ahead: Before you place the yogurt into the potatoes; you can chill the potatoes for up to one day. Reheat until they are hot. If they are stiff, add a small amount of milk until you reach the desired consistency.

Servings: 10 to 12

Soup

Egg & Lemon Greek Soup

Ingredients
¼ cup converted rice
½ teaspoon pepper
2 beaten eggs
6 cups chicken stock
1 teaspoon salt
Juice of 1 lemon

Preparation
1) Bring the chicken stock to simmer in a large pot. Blend in the rice and cook for 15 minutes.
2) Mix the lemon juice and eggs—slowly adding to the simmering broth.
3) Don't boil to prevent curdling.
4) The egg cooks instantly.
5) Flavor with pepper and salt.

Yields: 8 to 10 servings

Chapter 5: Dessert and Snack Recipes

Desserts

Ricotta Cheesecake

Ingredients
8 large eggs
3 pounds fresh ricotta cheese (whole milk)
Zest of 2 large oranges
½ pound or 1 cup sugar
Butter for coating the pan

Preparation
1) In a large container, blend all of the ingredients for around 10 minutes.
2) Use the butter to grease the entire inside of a ten-inch spring-form pan.
3) Empty the mix into the cake pan and bake at 425ºF for thirty minutes; reduce the temperature to 380ºF for an additional forty minutes.
4) Cool the cake and serve.

Almond Cake

Ingredients
6 large eggs (separated)

1 ¾ cups (1/2 pound) blanched whole almonds
1 ¼ cups superfine sugar
4 drops almond extract
Grated zest of 1 orange and 1 lemon
Dusting: Confectioner's sugar

Procedure

1) Use some butter to lightly grease an 11-inch spring-form pan, and drizzle it with flour to help prevent sticking.

2) Finely grind the almonds. A food processor is the easiest method.

3) Beat the sugar and egg yolks with an electric mixer for a pale, smooth cream.

4) Blend in the almond extract, the zests, and ground almonds. Mix well.

5) Using clean beaters whip the egg whites until stiff. Blend them into the almond and egg mixture.

6) Empty the batter into the greased spring-form pan and bake for 40 minutes.

7) Cool completely before moving it from the pan. The cake should be firm to the touch.

8) Garnish with the confectioner's sugar before serving.

Traditional Greek Yogurt Cake in Syrup

Ingredients
5 eggs (separated whites and yolks)
2 ¼ cups self-rising flour
1 cup yogurt
¾ cup butter (substitute ½ cup (+) 1 tablespoon olive oil)
1 1/8 cup sugar
3 tablespoons baking powder
1 teaspoon vanilla extract
Zest of 1 orange and 1 lemon

For the Syrup:
1 ½ cups sugar
½ teaspoon vanilla extract
1 ½ cups of water
3 to 4 tablespoons cognac

Procedure
1) Preheat the oven to 350ºF.

2) Put some oil on a cake pan approximately 10-inch (26cm) round cake tin to keep the cake from sticking.

3) In a small saucepan, prepare the syrup; combine all of the ingredients to a boil for two to three minutes. The syrup will slightly thicken.

4) For the cake, separate the eggs, and put the egg whites in the mixer with a dash of salt. Blend until it forms a thick peak (the meringues). Place it in a separate container and set to the side.

5) Use a mixing dish, combine the sugar and butter/oil with an electric mixer until the butter/oil is fluffy and creamy. Combine the egg yolks into the mixture, one-at-a-time, blending thoroughly each time. Toss in the lemon and orange zest, yogurt, and vanilla extract.

6) Blend in 1/3 of the sifted flour, blending with a maryse spatula from the bottom upwards. Continue with the remainder of the flour and meringue 1/3 each at a time.

7) Pour the batter into the baking pan, place it on the lower rack and bake 50 to 60 minutes.

8) Slowly, pour the cold syrup over the hot cake, letting each ladle soak into the cake before adding the next one.

The Greek cake is best-served cold with yogurt or fresh fruits.

Notes: Be sure the butter is at room temperature. Test the cake for doneness with a toothpick or wooden skewer. The stick should be clean if the cake is ready.

Yields: Serves 10 to 12

Grape Harvest Cake

Ingredients

- ½ cup ground almonds
- ¾ cup light brown sugar
- 2 tsp. baking powder
- ½ cup cornmeal
- ¾ cup all-purpose flour
- ½ tsp. salt

- 1/3 cup olive oil
- 2 cups red seedless grapes
- 1 tsp. almond extract
- 3 eggs
- ½ cup sour cream
- 1 Tbsp. each:
    - Brown sugar
    - White sugar

Preparation

1) Set the temperature of the oven to 350ºF.

2) Lightly grease a 9-inch spring-form pan with a bit of oil to prevent sticking.

3) Mix the baking powder, flour, cornmeal, salt, and ground almonds.

4) In another small dish, combine the almond extract, oil, and brown sugar. Blend in the eggs (1 at a time), and sour cream.

5) Blend in the flour mixture and mix thoroughly.

6) Bake 10 minutes, take the cake from the oven, and spread the grapes on top.

7) Blend the last sugars and garnish the top of the grapes.
8) Place in the oven and continue baking for about 30 to 35 additional minutes.
9) Cool the cake completely and enjoy!

Almond Coffee Cookies

Ingredients
50 whole coffee beans
1 tablespoon espresso ground coffee
1 pound almonds
Zest of 2 medium lemons
½ pound sugar
3 egg whites
2 tablespoons unsweetened cocoa powder
Glazing: ½ cup sugar

Procedure
1) Preheat the oven to 350ºF.
2) Boil the almonds to remove the peel and let them cool.
3) When the nuts are almost all of the way dry; place them in a blender/processor to chop them into a fine powder.

4) Place the almonds into a container; add the sugar, lemon zest, cocoa powder, and ground coffee. Blend well.

5) Add the eggs to the mixture until the almond mixture is a paste.

6) Roll each cookie into a ball smaller than a golf ball, and roll in in the sugar.

7) Place it on the cookie sheet and place a coffee bean on top of the cookie.

8) Roll them out and bake about 30 minutes.

Chocolate Chip-Oatmeal Raisin Cookies

Ingredients
1 ½ cups oatmeal (quick oats okay)
¾ cup buttermilk
1 tsp. cinnamon
1 cup shortening
¾ tsp. salt
2 beaten eggs
1 ½ cups brown sugar
1/2 tsp. cloves
½ cup chocolate chips
1 cup raisins

¾ cup teaspoon baking soda
2 cups flour

Preparation
1) Have a cookie sheet handy.
2) Blend the cinnamon, cloves, salt, and shortening.
3) Mix in the eggs and brown sugar to a cream texture.
4) Stir the raisins and oatmeal into the creamy mix.
5) Sift the baking soda and flour together and mix with the buttermilk.
6) Alternate the mixes until blended fully.
7) Drop by the spoon-full onto the prepared tray.
8) Bake approximately ten minutes.

Snacks or Appetizers

Cucumber Roll Ups

Ingredients
1 large cucumber
1/8 teaspoon black pepper

6 tablespoons each:
- Roasted red peppers
- Roasted garlic hummus
- Chopped sun-dried tomatoes
- Feta cheese crumbled

1 large cucumber

Preparation

1) Prepare the cucumber with a knife or veggie peeler to shave long, thin slices of cucumber. One cucumber will provide approximately 12 pieces.

2) Use a pinch of the black pepper on each slice.

3) Spread 1 ½ teaspoons of the feta and peppers on each slice.

4) Loosely roll the cucumber around the filling and close with a toothpick.

Serves 6

Pita Pizzas and Hummus

Ingredients
5 slices of pita bread

1 cup beef roast
½ cup artichokes
1 Can (10-ounces) whole tomatoes
½ cup chopped olives
10 tablespoons olive oil
½ lemon
1 tablespoon Tahini
1 cup chickpeas
1 cup Garbanzo beans
1 teaspoon oregano
½ cup feta cheese
To taste: Paprika and salt

Preparation
1) Preheat the oven to 250ºF.
2) Blend the can of tomatoes for the sauce.
3) Split the bread into halves on a baking tin.
4) On each slice, sprinkle a touch of oil along with 1 tablespoon of sauce.
5) Place the artichokes, roast beef, cheese, and black olives.
6) Top off with the salt and oregano.
7) Place the tray onto the broiler 5 minutes. Let it cool 3 or 4 minutes.

8) *For the Hummus*: Use a blender to combine 1 tablespoon of the Tahini, 1 tablespoon oil, salt, a pinch of paprika, ½ of a lemon, and1 cup each of the garbanzo and chickpeas.
9) Serve the hummus to side of the pizza for a healthier snack food.

Note: If the mixture for the hummus is too dry add a little more olive oil.

Mediterranean Skewers with Bloody Mary Vinaigrette

This is a delightful treat to be used as an appetizer or just to impress some friends and family!

Ingredients

- 2 celery hearts (3 tablespoons) diced fine
- ½ cup tomato juice
- ¼ teaspoon kosher salt

- 2 tablespoons premium vodka
- 1/8 teaspoon Worcestershire sauce
- ¼ teaspoon black pepper
- 2 tablespoons olive oil
- 1/8 teaspoon hot sauce
- ¼ teaspoon prepared horseradish
- Grape tomatoes
- Bocconcini
- Kalamata Olives (approximately 32)
- Artichoke Hearts

Preparation
1) In a medium dish, combine the vodka, tomato juice, hot sauce, Worcestershire, oil, horseradish, pepper, and salt. Place in the fridge.
2) Each skewer should have a Bocconcini ball, artichoke, tomato, and olive.
3) Serve the skewers with vinaigrette.

How easy is that?

Notes: In case you are not sure, Bocconcini is a small portion of mozzarella cheeses which are in the size of an egg.

Yields: 32 servings = 1 skewer + 1 ½ teaspoons vinaigrette

Cranberry, Goat Cheese, and Walnut Canapés

Ingredients
24 slices (thin) whole wheat baguette (from 1/2 baguette)
¾ cup (approximately 24 halves) walnuts
Ground pepper and coarse salt
1/8 teaspoon ground cinnamon
4 teaspoons olive oil
½ cup dried cranberries
8 ounces fresh goat cheese
1 teaspoon fresh chopped thyme (+) leaves for garnishing

Preparation
1) Preset the oven temperature to 375ºF.

2) Use a baking sheet with high sides; place 1 teaspoon oil, salt, pepper, and cinnamon—toss in the nuts.

3) Bake 4 to 6 minutes. Set to the side.

4) Using the same sheet, place the baguette slices and brush with oil, flavoring with pepper and salt.

5) Bake for 10 to 15 minutes. Rotate the pan ½ through the cooking process.

6) In a medium bowl, blend 2 tablespoons water with the cheese. Blend in the thyme and cranberries with a dash of pepper or salt.

Serve the goat cheese among the slices of bread. Garnish each one with thyme leaves and walnut.

Greek Yogurt Parfait

Ingredients
¼ cup unsalted dry roasted pistachios
3 cups plain yogurt
4 teaspoons honey
1 teaspoon vanilla extract

28 clementine segments

Preparation

1) Shell and chop the pistachios.

2) Blend the vanilla and yogurt in a dish. (Greek-style fat-free is the best choice.)

3) Spoon approximately 1/3 cup of the yogurt blend into four parfait glasses (the bottom layer).

4) Garnish each with five clementine sections, ½ teaspoon honey, and ½ tablespoon of the nuts.

5) Use the remainder of the yogurt mix in each of the cups—topping each off with ½ tablespoon of the nuts, ½ teaspoon of the honey, and 2 each of the clementine sections.

Enjoy immediately!

Yields: 1 parfait = 4 servings

Note: The clementine is a cross between a sweet orange and a mandarin orange.

Yogurt and Honey with Walnuts: Greek-Style

Ingredients
1 ½ to 2 cups toasted walnuts
2 to 3 cups plain yogurt
½ to ¾ cup honey
¾ to 1 teaspoon vanilla

Preparation
1) Blend the vanilla and yogurt
2) Layer the ingredients between the glasses.
3) Start with yogurt and polish it off with the walnuts and honey.
What a treat!

Servings: 4 to 6

Lemon Cream & Blueberries

Ingredients
1 teaspoon honey
¾ cup low-fat vanilla yogurt

4 ounces reduced-fat cream cheese
2 cups fresh blueberries
2 teaspoons lemon zest (freshly grated)

Preparation

1) Drain the liquid from the yogurt, and use a fork to break up the cheese into a dish. Combine the mixture and the honey, and blend with an electric mixer at the highest speed until creamy and light.
2) Blend in the lemon zest.
3) Layer the blueberries and cream in dessert dishes.

Note: If you want to serve it later, refrigerate it for up to a maximum of 8 hours in an air-tight container.

Chapter 6: Continue the Plan

You now have some of the information necessary to get your health back in line and feel better in the process. This chapter will provide you with some basic guidelines that will be useful for your continued success with the Mediterranean diet plan. The following guideline for meal plans is to guide you through your journey. Try out some of the tempting recipes for breakfast, lunch, and dinner. Each of the recipes contained in this book is delicious.

Sample Meal Plan

You have got the basis for your meal plan; these will assist you on the days when you aren't sure what you want to have on the menu for the day.

Monday
A veggie omelet with onions and tomatoes and a piece of fruit
A whole grain sandwich with cheese; fresh veggies on the side
Mediterranean Lasagna

Tuesday
Oatmeal with raisins
Tuna salad
Salad with olives, tomatoes, and feta cheese

Wednesday
Oatmeal with nuts and raisins with an apple
Who grain sandwich with veggies
Mediterranean pizza made from whole wheat garnished with cheese, olives, and other veggies

Thursday
Eggs and veggies fried in olive oil
Greek yogurt with nuts, oats, and strawberries
Grilled lamb with baked potato and a salad

Friday
Omelet with olives and vegetables
Pizza
Grilled chicken with potatoes and veggies; fruit for dessert

Saturday
Greek yogurt with oats and strawberries
Veggies with a whole grain sandwich
Tuna salad and a piece of fruit

Sunday
Yogurt with nuts and sliced fruits
Leftover *Beef Steaks Crusted in Cumin with Olive-Orange Relish* from the night before
Broiled salmon with veggies and brown rice

Healthy Snacks

- Leftovers from dinner
- A piece of fruit
- Splurge/Apple slices with almond butter

- Berries or grapes
- Greek yogurt
- A handful of nuts
- Carrots

How to Eat Out and Remain on the Diet

1) Have seafood or fish as your main dish.
2) Eat only whole grain bread with olive oil. Do not use butter.
3) Request your food be cooked using extra-virgin olive oil.

The Substitution List

This is a short list of ways to help maintain your diet as a general outline:

- Instead of crackers, pretzels, chips, and ranch dip; try some celery, carrots, broccoli and salsa.
- Leave the white rice and stir-fried meat behind and replace it with some quinoa with stir-fried veggies.

- So, you really want that big dish of ice cream; leave it and have some budding made with skim or whole milk.

Myths about the Plan

Myth #1: The Mediterranean diet is just another food plan.
Fact #1: The Mediterranean diet is a good food plan, but the plan helps in many other ways as have been indicated in this report/book. The food is made to be enjoyed in a relaxed atmosphere which is equally important to your health as to what is on your plate

Myth #2: Have a huge bowl of pasta and bread; it is the Mediterranean way!
Fact #2: Pasta is usually a side dish with the Mediterranean culture; they do not eat like the Americans. The helping is generally a portion of ½-cup to 1-cup. Most of the meal consists of fish, vegetables, and salads; sometimes—a slice of bread or some grass-fed meat.

Myth #3: It is expensive to eat on this plan.
Fact #3: The Mediterranean plan is not expensive if you are making the creation from lentils and beans for the protein source. You are also sticking with the whole grains and mostly plants which are much cheaper than the processed or prepackaged food items.

Myth #4: Three glasses of wine are great since one is good for your heart.
Fact #4: The diet plan allows some red wines in moderation which means two for men and one drink for women daily. Over those limits, can be damaging for your heart, health, and well-being.

Conclusion

It is my sincere hope that you might have liked all the recipes which have been mentioned in the book and once again thank you for getting this book and experimenting with the recipes.

About The Author

Jimmy Morris is born with the vision to promote *Intermittent fasting* among the masses. The author has written several research papers on the topic. He has served as an instructor promoting various cultural arts in University of San Francisco. He is currently living with his spouse in Texas.

www.ingramcontent.com/pod-product-compliance
Lightning Source LLC
LaVergne TN
LVHW011943070526
838202LV00054B/4774